Global Health

Editor: Danielle Lobban

Volume 419

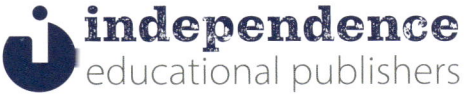

First published by Independence Educational Publishers

The Studio, High Green

Great Shelford

Cambridge CB22 5EG

England

© Independence 2023

Copyright

This book is sold subject to the condition that it shall not, by way of trade or otherwise, be lent, resold, hired out or otherwise circulated in any form of binding or cover other than that in which it is published without the publisher's prior consent.

Photocopy licence

The material in this book is protected by copyright. However, the purchaser is free to make multiple copies of particular articles for instructional purposes for immediate use within the purchasing institution. Making copies of the entire book is not permitted.

ISBN-13: 978 1 86168 879 8

Printed in Great Britain

Zenith Print Group

Acknowledgements

The publisher is grateful for permission to reproduce the material in this book. While every care has been taken to trace and acknowledge copyright, the publisher tenders its apology for any accidental infringement or where copyright has proved untraceable. The publisher would be pleased to come to a suitable arrangement in any such case with the rightful owner.

The material reproduced in **issues** books is provided as an educational resource only. The views, opinions and information contained within reprinted material in **issues** books do not necessarily represent those of Independence Educational Publishers and its employees.

Images

Cover image courtesy of iStock. All other images courtesy of Freepik, Pixabay and Unsplash.

Additional acknowledgements

With thanks to the Independence team: Shelley Baldry, Tracy Biram, Klaudia Sommer and Jackie Staines.

Danielle Lobban

Cambridge, January 2023

Contents

Chapter 1: Global Health Issues

The 13 biggest threats to global health, according to WHO	1
What is the difference between pandemic, endemic, and epidemic?	4
10 Pandemics throughout history	6
The impact of COVID-19 on global health goals	8
What to know about coronaviruses	12
The recent monkeypox outbreak is a reminder that our interconnected world has its dangers	14
Ebola: what are the symptoms, how does it spread and where did it come from?	15
Ebola outbreak re-ignites debate over international travel checks in UK and US	17
World Malaria Report 2021 – A more accurate picture of the malaria burden in Africa	19
What is malaria?	20
New malaria vaccine comes a step closer as experts say it's 'the best yet'	22
How climate change is amplifying mosquito-borne diseases	24
Antimicrobial resistance now causes more deaths than HIV/AIDS and malaria worldwide – new study	26
What is antimicrobial resistance and why do we need to take action against it?	28

Chapter 2: Future Health

UK 'no better prepared for the next pandemic' with 'dangerous gaps' in its health security	30
How can the world handle the next pandemic if it struggles with new variants?	32
From cholera to COVID: a brief history of vaccines	34
Scientists around the world are already fighting the next pandemic	37
Useful Websites	42
Glossary	42
Index	44

Introduction

Global Health is Volume 419 in the issues series. The aim of the series is to offer current, diverse information about important issues in our world, from a UK perspective.

About Global Health

Advances in medicine and technology over the past few years have increased the general health of people around the world. This book explores some of the health issues that affect people around the globe and the methods used to try to prevent and treat these issues.

Our sources

Titles in the issues series are designed to function as educational resource books, providing a balanced overview of a specific subject.

The information in our books is comprised of facts, articles and opinions from many different sources, including:

- Newspaper reports and opinion pieces
- Website factsheets
- Magazine and journal articles
- Statistics and surveys
- Government reports
- Literature from special interest groups.

A note on critical evaluation

Because the information reprinted here is from a number of different sources, readers should bear in mind the origin of the text and whether the source is likely to have a particular bias when presenting information (or when conducting their research). It is hoped that, as you read about the many aspects of the issues explored in this book, you will critically evaluate the information presented.

It is important that you decide whether you are being presented with facts or opinions. Does the writer give a biased or unbiased report? If an opinion is being expressed, do you agree with the writer? Is there potential bias to the 'facts' or statistics behind an article?

Activities

Throughout this book, you will find a selection of assignments and activities designed to help you engage with the articles you have been reading and to explore your own opinions. Some tasks will take longer than others and there is a mixture of design, writing and research-based activities that you can complete alone or in a group.

Further research

At the end of each article we have listed its source and a website that you can visit if you would like to conduct your own research. Please remember to critically evaluate any sources that you consult and consider whether the information you are viewing is accurate and unbiased.

Issues Online

The **issues** series of books is complemented by our online resource, issuesonline.co.uk

On the Issues Online website you will find a wealth of information, covering over 70 topics, to support the PSHE and RSE curriculum.

Why Issues Online?

Researching a topic? Issues Online is the best place to start for...

Librarians

Issues Online is an essential tool for librarians: feel confident you are signposting safe, reliable, user-friendly online resources to students and teaching staff alike. We provide multi-user concurrent access, so no waiting around for another student to finish with a resource. Issues Online also provides FREE downloadable posters for your shelf/wall/table displays.

Teachers

Issues Online is an ideal resource for lesson planning, inspiring lively debate in class and setting homework tasks.

Our accessible, engaging content helps deepen students knowledge, promotes critical thinking and develops independent learning skills.

Issues Online saves precious preparation time. We wade through the wealth of material on the internet to filter the best quality, most relevant and up-to-date information you need to start exploring a topic.

Our carefully selected, balanced content presents an overview and insight into each topic from a variety of sources and viewpoints.

Students

Issues Online is designed to support your studies in a broad range of topics, particularly social issues relevant to young people today.

Thousands of articles, statistics and infographs instantly available to help you with research and assignments.

With 24/7 access using the powerful Algolia search system, you can find relevant information quickly, easily and safely anytime from your laptop, tablet or smartphone, in class or at home.

Visit www.issuesonline.co.uk for more information

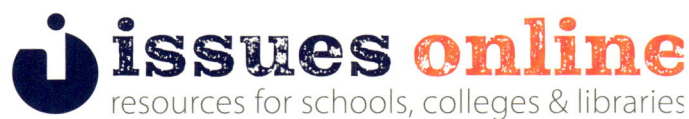

Chapter 1

Global Health Issues

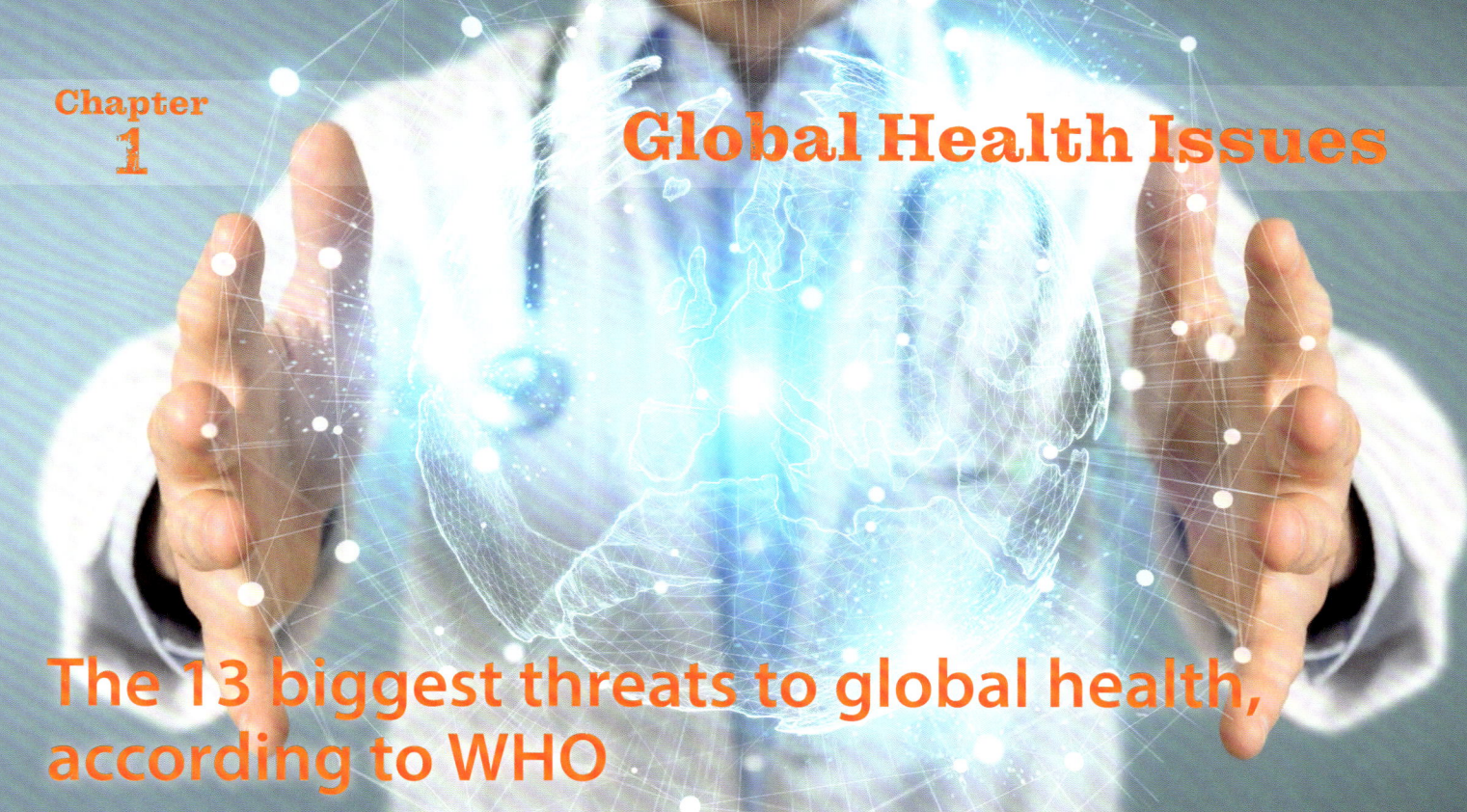

The 13 biggest threats to global health, according to WHO

The World Health Organization (WHO) recently released a list of 13 urgent health challenges the world will face over next decade, which highlights a range of issues including climate change and health care equity.

About the list

According to WHO, the list provides an overview of 'urgent, global health challenges' that WHO developed with help from experts around the world. WHO said the challenges included on the list 'demand a response from more than just the health sector,' adding, 'Governments, communities, and international agencies must work together' to address these 'critical' issues.

WHO said all of the challenges included on the list are urgent, and several are interlinked. As such, WHO did not list the challenges in any particular order.

The 13 biggest health challenges for the next decade

1. Climate crisis

The world's climate crisis has major health implications, according to WHO, with air pollution alone killing an estimated seven million people annually. In addition, more than 25% of deaths from chronic respiratory disease, heart attack, lung cancer, and stroke are attributed to the same emissions responsible for global warming, WHO said. Climate change also worsens malnutrition and promotes the spread of infectious diseases, according to WHO.

To address the issue, WHO said it is working toward creating 'a set of policy options for governments' that aim to lower the health risks associated with air pollution. The organization said, 'Leaders in both the public and private sectors must work together to clean up our air and mitigate the health impacts of climate change.'

2. Health care delivery in areas of conflict and crisis

WHO noted that, in 2019, most of the disease outbreaks that required the organization's 'highest level of … response occurred in countries with protracted conflicts.' WHO said it recorded a total of 978 attacks against health care workers or facilities in 11 countries last year, which resulted in 193 deaths. The conflicts also forced a record number of people to leave their homes, resulting in limited health care access for tens of millions of people, WHO said.

WHO noted that it is 'working with countries and partners to strengthen health systems, improve preparedness, and expand the availability of long-term contingency financing for complex health emergencies.' However, the group said 'political solutions' are need 'to resolve protracted conflicts, stop neglecting the weakest health systems, and protect health care workers and facilities from attacks.'

3. Health care equity

There are major discrepancies in the quality of people's health across socio-economic groups, WHO said. For example, WHO noted that there is an 18-year difference between the life expectancy of people in low- and high-income countries, as well as significant differences in life expectancies among people living within the same countries and cities. In addition, low- and middle-income countries face a disproportionately large burden of cancer, diabetes, and other noncommunicable diseases, which can quickly put a strain on the resources of low-income households.

WHO said it is working to address disparities in health equity by improving 'child and maternal care, nutrition, gender equality, mental health, and access to adequate water and sanitation' and providing guidance on how countries can work to improve health care equity.

4. Access to treatments

According to WHO, about one-third of people across the world lack access to essential health products such as diagnostic tools, medicines, and vaccines. Limited access to these products fuel drug resistance and threaten people's lives and health, according to WHO.

To address the issue, WHO said it will 'sharpen its focus' on efforts to combat 'substandard and falsified medical products; enhance the capacity of low-income countries to assure the quality of medical products throughout the supply chain; and improve access to diagnosis and treatment for noncommunicable diseases.'

5. Infectious disease prevention

HIV, sexually transmitted infections, viral hepatitis and other infectious diseases will kill an estimated four million people this year, accord to WHO. Vaccine-preventable diseases also are expected to kill thousands of people over the next decade.

Part of the reason why infectious diseases continue to spread is because of weak health systems in endemic countries and insufficient levels of financing, WHO said. As such, WHO said there is 'an urgent need for greater political will and increased funding for essential health services; strengthening routine immunization; improving the quality and availability of data to inform planning, and more efforts to mitigate the effects of drug resistance.'

6. Epidemic preparedness

An airborne and highly infectious virus pandemic 'is inevitable,' WHO said, but countries around the world continue to spend more on responding to these emergencies than preparing for them. This leaves countries unprepared for when another pandemic strikes and potentially threatens the lives of millions of people, according to WHO.

WHO said countries should invest in evidence-based practices to strengthen their health systems and protect populations from disease outbreaks, natural disasters, and other health emergencies.

7. Unsafe products

Nearly one-third of today's global disease burden is attributed to a lack of food, unsafe food, and unhealthy diets, according to WHO. WHO said while food insecurity and hunger continue to be an issue, there also is a growing number of people who have diets that are high in fat or sugar, leading to a rise in weight- and diet-related diseases. Further, there's been an increase in tobacco and e-cigarette use in most countries, raising additional health concerns.

WHO said it is looking to combat health risks related to unsafe foods and other products by 'working with countries to develop evidence-based public policies, investments, and private sector reforms to reshape food systems and provide healthy and sustainable diets,' and 'to build political

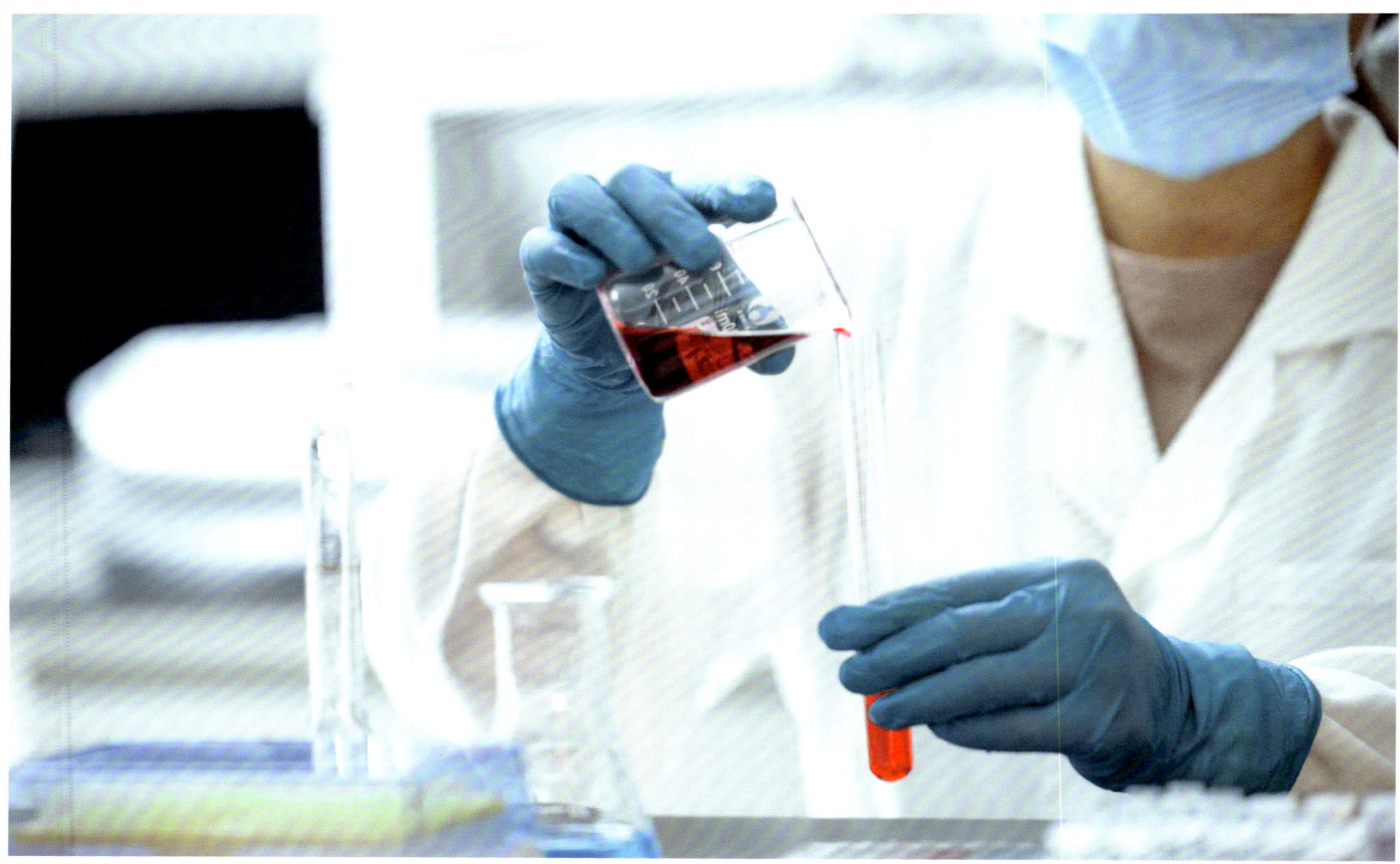

commitment and capacity to strengthen implementation of evidence-based tobacco control policies.'

8. Underinvestment in health workers

There is a shortage of health workers around the world because of low pay and chronic underinvestment in health workers' education and employment, WHO said. According to WHO, the shortages negatively affect health systems' sustainability and jeopardize health and social care services. An additional 18 million health workers, including nine million nurses and midwives, will be needed across the world by 2030, according to WHO.

WHO said the World Health Assembly has designated 2020 as the 'Year of the Nurse and the Midwife' in an effort to spur 'action and encourage investment in education, skills, and jobs' for health care workers. In addition, WHO said it is working with countries to generate new investments to ensure health care workers are trained and paid 'decent salaries.'

9. Adolescent safety

Each year, more than one million adolescents ages 10 to 19 die, with road injuries, HIV, suicide, lower respiratory infections, and interpersonal violence leading as causes of death among teens. According to WHO, a number of factors—including harmful alcohol use, unprotected sex, and lack of physical activity—increase the risks of these types of death.

WHO said it will aim to promote mental health and curb harmful behaviours among adolescents in 2020 by issuing new guidance and working to bolster emergency trauma care.

10. Improving public trust of health care workers

The spread of misinformation, coupled with weakening trust of public institutions, is playing an increasing role in the health decisions patients make, according to WHO. But when patients trust health care systems, they are more likely to follow a health care worker's advice on how to stay healthy and are more likely to rely on health services, WHO said.

In order to bolster public trust in health care workers and systems, WHO said it is working to help countries 'strengthen primary care' and to combat misinformation on social media platforms. Further, WHO added that 'scientists and the public health community need to do a better job of listening to the communities they serve,' and there is a need for investments 'in better public health data information systems.'

11. Capitalizing on technological advancements

Breakthroughs in technology have revolutionized disease diagnosis, prevention, and treatment, WHO said, and genome editing, digital health technologies, and synthetic biology have the potential to solve a number of health problems.

However, WHO also noted that these technologies raise a number of questions regarding how they should be regulated and monitored. WHO cautioned that without the appropriate guardrails, these technological advancements have the potential to create new organisms and harm people, and said it is setting up new advisory committees to review evidence and provide guidance on the technologies.

12. Threat of anti-microbial resistance and other medicines

Anti-microbial resistance (AMR) has the potential to undo decades of medical advancements and has increased due to a number of factors, including limited access to quality and low-cost medications, the unregulated prescription and use of antibiotics, poor infection control, and more, WHO said.

The organization said it is working to combat AMR 'by addressing its root causes, while advocating for research and development into new antibiotics.'

13. Health care sanitation

Billions of people across the world live in communities without adequate sanitation services or potable water, which are major causes of disease. And about one-fourth of health care facilities across the world lack basic water services, which are critical to health systems, WHO said. A lack of water and other basic resources results in poor-quality care and increases the likelihood of infections, according to WHO.

To address the issue, WHO and its partners are working with low- and middle-income countries to improve hygiene, sanitation, and water conditions at the countries' health care facilities. WHO also is calling on all countries to ensure all health care facilities have basic hygiene, sanitation, and water services by 2030 (WHO, 'Urgent health challenges for the next decade,' 1/13).

15 January 2020

Consider...

This article was written at the beginning of the Covid-19 pandemic. How do you think the global health threats have changed since then?

Design

Choose one of the 13 global health threats and design a poster to create awareness of the situation.

The above information is reprinted with kind permission from Advisory Board.
© 2023 Advisory Board

www.advisory.com

What is the difference between pandemic, endemic, and epidemic?

Pandemic, endemic, and epidemic are all terms that describe how far a disease or pathogen has spread within a geographical region or population.

Medically reviewed by Joseph Vinetz, MD

By: Caitlin Geng

An endemic disease is one that is always present throughout a region or group of people and remains fairly consistent. An example of this is coccidioidomycosis, or valley fever, which is endemic to the Southwestern United States and northern Mexico.

An epidemic occurs when a disease unexpectedly increases among a large population or region. An example is ebola, which spread rapidly throughout West Africa in 2014–2016.

A pandemic spreads across multiple countries or continents, affecting large numbers of people. An example of this is COVID-19, which results from a coronavirus called SARS-CoV-2 that first appeared in one region before spreading around the world.

In this article, we look at the differences between pandemic, endemic, and epidemic diseases. We also give more examples of each and explain which is most severe.

What does 'endemic' mean?

An endemic disease is one that is always present throughout a specific region or population. The prevalence of the disease remains fairly stable and predictable over time.

Some examples of endemic conditions include:

- Malaria: This mosquito-borne illness is present in many countries worldwide. However, it is endemic to parts of Africa, among other places, because the higher temperatures allow the Anopheles mosquito, which spreads malaria, to thrive. This means that malaria remains at constant levels in this region.
- Coccidioidomycosis: Inhaling fungal spores causes this condition, which is also known as valley fever. It is endemic to the Southwestern U.S. and northern Mexico.
- Dengue fever: This condition is endemic to tropical and subtropical regions because, as with malaria, it spreads through mosquito bites. The Aedes mosquito carries viruses that can cause dengue fever.
- Hepatitis B: The hepatitis B virus (HBV) is endemic worldwide, although it has higher endemicity in Africa and Asia than in Europe and North America. HBV spreads through contact with blood that contains the virus. Due to this, it does not cause the sudden outbreaks that airborne viruses can.

What is an epidemic?

An epidemic occurs when a disease spreads unexpectedly or quickly across a geographical area or population. It can occur if an endemic disease suddenly becomes more prevalent, or if a new disease begins to affect a region or group.

Many examples of epidemics involve contagious illnesses, but there are exceptions.

Some examples of epidemics include:

- Zika virus: Scientists first identified this mosquito-borne virus in monkeys in 1947. Zika virus began affecting humans in the 1950s, but it did not cause its first outbreak until 2007. In 2014, it caused an outbreak in Polynesia and then Brazil. From here, it quickly spread to the Caribbean and most of South America.
- Ebola virus: There have been several outbreaks of ebola in various African nations since the 1970s, but in 2013, it became an epidemic in West Africa.
- Opioids: In the U.S., the use of opioids has increased dramatically in recent decades, causing a substantial increase in overdoses. Between 1999 and 2019, there were nearly 500,000 deaths due to opioid overdose. Many more people have ongoing addictions to these substances, which include prescription medication and recreational drugs, such as heroin.

What is a pandemic?

A pandemic occurs when a disease spreads across countries or continents. Scientists may determine that a disease has become a pandemic if it spreads at a very fast rate, with new cases appearing every day.

Pandemics have become more likely due to international travel. People travel to different countries and continents more often than before. Greater urbanization also means that many people live in densely populated towns and cities. This proximity allows the rapid transmission of pathogens from person to person.

Changes in how people use land and exploit the natural environment also play a role. Several pandemics from the past few decades have been zoonotic diseases, which means that they result from viruses that originally affected a species of animal.

However, close contact between animals and humans increases the likelihood of such viruses evolving and adapting to infect humans, too. Some examples of activities that increase the chance of this include:

- keeping livestock
- hunting or trading wild animals
- eating wild animals

Some examples of pandemics include:

- Bubonic plague: The bubonic plague, also known as the 'Black Death,' spreads through flea bites. A bacterium known as Yersinia pestis causes it. The bubonic plague became a pandemic in the 14th century. The disease still exists today and is most endemic in Madagascar, the Democratic Republic of the Congo, and Peru. It is also present in the U.S., particularly in the southwestern states, which include Arizona and Colorado.
- 1918 influenza: A specific strain of influenza (flu) virus caused this pandemic. It affected more than one-third of the global population in 1918 and caused about 50 million deaths.
- HIV: This virus attacks the immune system, making people vulnerable to many other infections. Experts believe that HIV came from chimpanzees before transmitting to humans. This transmission may have happened as early as the late 19th century. HIV reached the United States in the mid-to-late 1970s.
- Severe acute respiratory syndrome (SARS): A virus known as SARS-CoV-1 causes this disease. Experts first identified the virus in Asia in 2003. SARS spread to more than 24 countries in various continents before international efforts to contain it proved successful.
- Swine flu: The H1N1 virus causes swine flu. The first known cases of swine flu in the U.S. were in 2009. The virus, which contains a unique combination of influenza genes that scientists had never seen before, spread across the globe, causing an estimated 151,700–575,400 fatalities worldwide.
- COVID-19: The SARS-CoV-2 virus causes this disease, which experts first detected in late 2019. Many scientists believe that it originated in a wild animal before transmitting to humans, although the exact origin is unclear.

Which is worse?

The terms 'pandemic,' 'epidemic,' and 'endemic' do not describe the severity of a disease. Instead, they describe its prevalence. This means that one is not inherently worse than the other.

For example, it is possible for an endemic illness to devastate communities and economies. The term indicates that the level of disease remains steady, rather than the number of cases.

It is also possible to have mild pandemics, in which an illness travels rapidly to many regions but does not cause severe illness or death. In contrast, an epidemic could be severe, causing significant illness and death in most of the people whom it affects.

What someone considers to be the worst depends on what they are measuring. In terms of scale, pandemics are the largest and have the biggest potential to cause worldwide disruption. Whether they fulfil this potential depends on the disease and how humans respond to it.

Can an epidemic become a pandemic?

An endemic disease can become an epidemic or pandemic, and vice versa.

An example of this is cholera. This illness occurs when a person swallows water or food containing Vibrio cholerae bacteria. It originated in India, but in the 19th century, it caused an outbreak that ultimately spread across the globe.

This cholera pandemic was the first of seven. The seventh, which still affects South Asia, Africa, and the Americas, is ongoing.

However, in many places, cholera has become endemic. This means that it is constantly present at relatively steady levels. Epidemics can also occur, even in locations without endemic cholera.

An endemic disease is not necessarily inevitable, and action may still be necessary to stop it. Cholera, for example, is a treatable and preventable disease. Clean water, sanitation, rehydration treatment, and vaccines can easily prevent many of the deaths that cholera currently causes.

Summary

Endemic, epidemic, and pandemic are all terms that scientists use to categorize diseases in terms of how widespread they are.

An endemic condition is one that is constant among a population or area, while an epidemic is a sudden spike in cases in one population or location. A pandemic is similar, but it spreads farther, affecting multiple regions or continents.

The severity of a disease depends on several factors. Due to this, although a pandemic affects a higher number of people, it is not necessarily more lethal than an epidemic or an endemic disease.

25 February 2022

The above information is reprinted with kind permission from Medical News Today. Republished from What is the difference between pandemic, endemic, and epidemic? by Caitlin Geng by permission of Medical News Today.

© 2004-2022 Healthline Media UK Ltd, Brighton, UK, a Red Ventures Company

www.medicalnewstoday.com

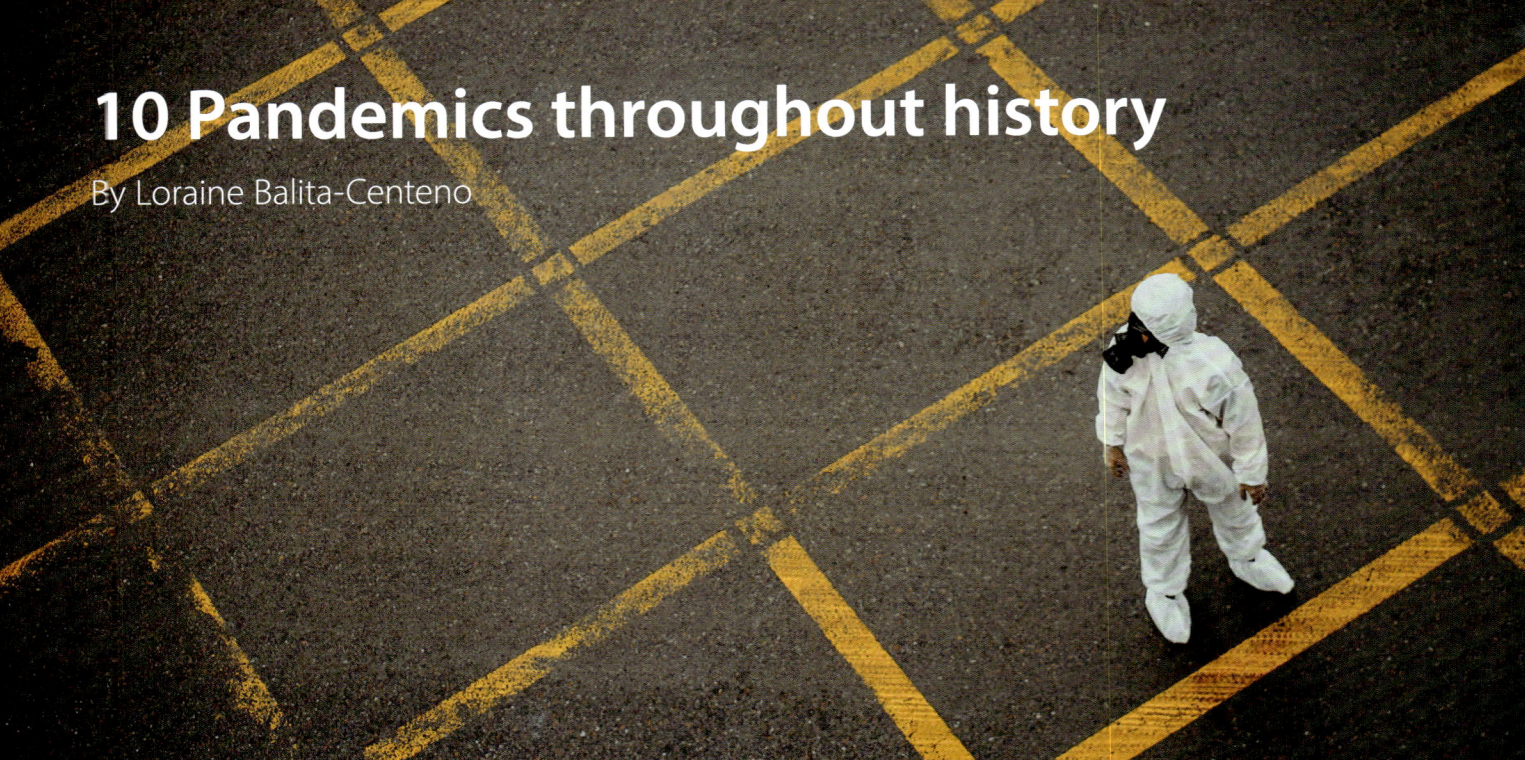

10 Pandemics throughout history

By Loraine Balita-Centeno

The coronavirus pandemic isn't the first to hit the human civilization. Throughout history there have been numerous pandemics, others much worse than COVID-19, that claimed the lives of thousands even millions of people. Ever since humans learned to live in groups forming communities where they live close to each other and also travel across the seas, the world has seen numerous diseases spread like wildfire. Here are ten pandemics that plagued humans in the past.

10. Antonine Plague (165 AD-180 AD)

Also known as the Plague of Galen, it was an ancient pandemic that broke out across the Roman Empire, through Asia, all Roman cities in Italy, and Greece. Eventually, it reached Spain, Egypt, and North Africa among other areas. At the height of the pandemic, it killed 2,000 people per day. Many believe that it was caused by smallpox and measles.

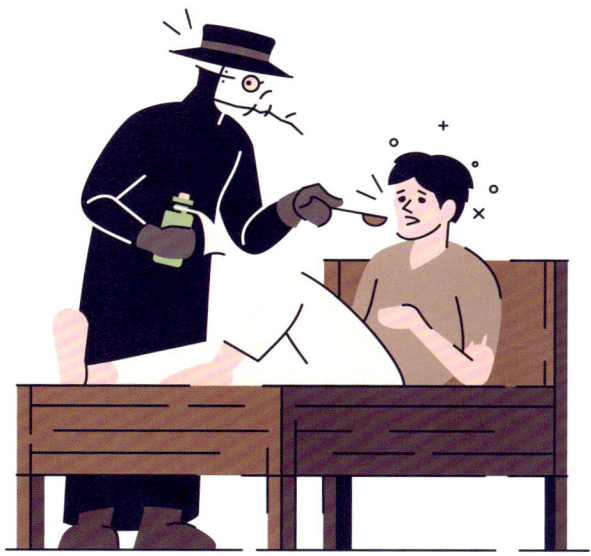

9. The Black Death (1347-1352)

It was the deadly pandemic that swept through Europe and Asia among other continents and killed an estimated 25 million people in Europe. Aside from having fever and chills, those afflicted also had blood and pus seeping out of swellings all over the body.

8. Smallpox Pandemic (1870-1874)

Before the world completely rid itself of this horrendous disease, it swept through continents killing three out of ten victims. Those who survived were left with deep scars which were even found in 3000-year-old mummies, showing that it ravaged ancient civilizations for thousands of years. But it was in 1870 during the Franco-Prussian war that smallpox spread throughout the world. From Europe, it reached Asia through America causing 500,000 deaths worldwide.

7. Cholera (1871-1824)

The first of seven cholera pandemics emerged in India in 1817. According to the World Health Organization cholera is an acute diarrheal infection caused by the ingestion of food or water contaminated with the bacterium Vibrio cholerae. Three years after it spread throughout India it reached different countries in Asia. In 1821 it was brought by British troops traveling from India even to countries outside Asia.

6. Russian Flu of 1889 (1889-1890)

Called the first-ever modern flu pandemic, the Russian flu which started in St. Petersburg, spread through Europe infecting even prominent world leaders. After a few months, it reached virtually every part of the planet. An estimated 1 million people died of the Russian flu.

5. Spanish Flu (1918-1919)

The Spanish Flu of 1918 is considered the deadliest in history, infecting 1/3 of the world's population and killing 20 to 50 million people worldwide. It came in three waves. The first wave was almost like the common flu and hit in the spring of 1918. The second wave that appeared in the fall of the same year was deadlier. It killed people within hours or a few days after the onset of symptoms. The third wave that came the following year was just as deadly and added more to the death toll.

4. H3N2 Pandemic (1968)

The 1968 flu pandemic was caused by the influenza H3N2 virus. Although relatively not as deadly, the virus was highly contagious that it spread throughout Southeast Asia within two weeks after it first emerged in Hong Kong in July 1968. By December the virus has reached The United States, United Kingdom, and other countries in Europe. It killed an estimated one million people.

3. HIV/AIDS (1981)

The first case of acquired immunodeficiency syndrome (AIDS) was reported in 1981. Since then HIV (Human Immunodeficiency Virus) has spread globally infecting more than 65 million people according to the Centers for Disease Control and Prevention. There is still no known cure for this sexually transmitted disease but there are already treatments that keep the virus under control allowing people to live longer.

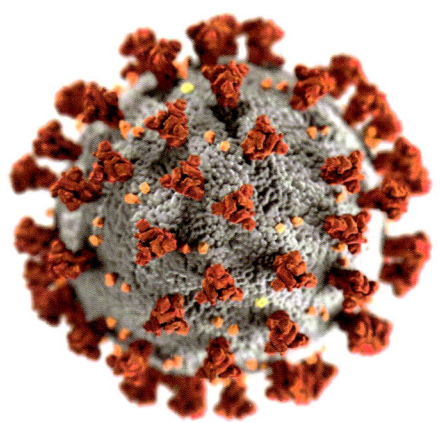

2. SARS (2002-2004)

Severe Acute Respiratory Syndrome (SARS) was first reported in Guangdong, China in February 2003 although experts believe it started in China as early as November 2002. After a few months, it spread throughout countries in North America, South America, Europe, and Asia. It infected 8,098 people worldwide and killed 774 people. The disease caused high fever, body aches, and dry cough which then led to pneumonia in some cases.

1. COVID-19 Pandemic 2019

Coronavirus is believed to have originated in Wuhan in China, the virus spread throughout Europe, the rest of Asia, North America and virtually every part of the world within months since it emerged in late 2019. It inflicted over 2 million people and killed hundreds of thousands worldwide.

14 April 2020

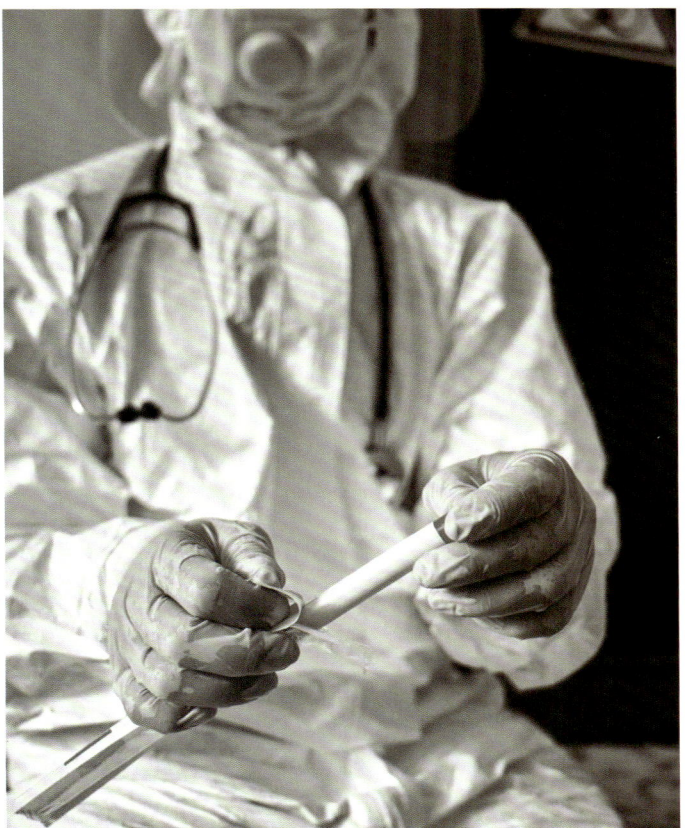

Key Facts

- Smallpox was declared eradicated in 1980 following a global immunization program led by the World Health Organization.

- Severe acute respiratory syndrome (SARS) is a viral respiratory illness caused by a coronavirus called SARS-associated coronavirus (SARS-CoV).

- According to the CDC, cholera, caused by the bacteria Vibrio cholerae, is rare in the United States and other industrialized nations.

The above information is reprinted with kind permission from worldatlas.com
© 2023 worldatlas.com

www.worldatlas.com

The impact of COVID-19 on global health goals

COVID-19 responsible for at least 3 million excess deaths in 2020.

As of 31 December 2020, COVID-19 had infected over 82 million people and killed more than 1.8 million worldwide. But preliminary estimates suggest the total number of global 'excess deaths' directly and indirectly attributable to COVID-19 in 2020 amount to at least 3 million, 1.2 million higher than the official figures reported by countries to WHO.

COVID-19 global excess mortality

While 1,813,188 COVID-19 deaths were reported in 2020, recent WHO estimates suggest an excess mortality of at least 3,000,000.

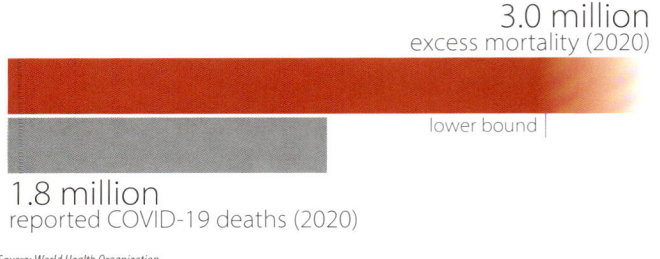

3.0 million excess mortality (2020)

lower bound

1.8 million reported COVID-19 deaths (2020)

Source: World Health Organization

With the latest COVID-19 deaths reported to WHO now exceeding 3.3 million, based on the estimates produced for 2020, we are likely facing a significant undercount of total deaths directly and indirectly attributed to COVID-19.

The term 'excess deaths' describes deaths beyond what would have been expected under 'normal' conditions. It captures not only confirmed deaths, but also COVID-19 deaths that were not correctly diagnosed and reported as well as deaths attributable to the overall crisis conditions. This provides a more comprehensive and accurate measure when compared with confirmed COVID-19 deaths alone.

> **The COVID-19 pandemic has shown the importance of data and science to build back more resilient health systems and equitably accelerate towards our shared global goals.**
> – Dr Tedros Adhanom Ghebreyesus

For example, some countries only report COVID-19 deaths occurring in hospitals or the deaths of people who have tested positive for COVID-19. In addition, many countries cannot accurately measure or report cause of death due to inadequate or under-resourced health information systems.

The pandemic has likely increased deaths from other causes due to disruption to health service delivery and routine immunizations, fewer people seeking care, and shortages

As household overcrowding increases, preventative COVID-19 behaviours decrease

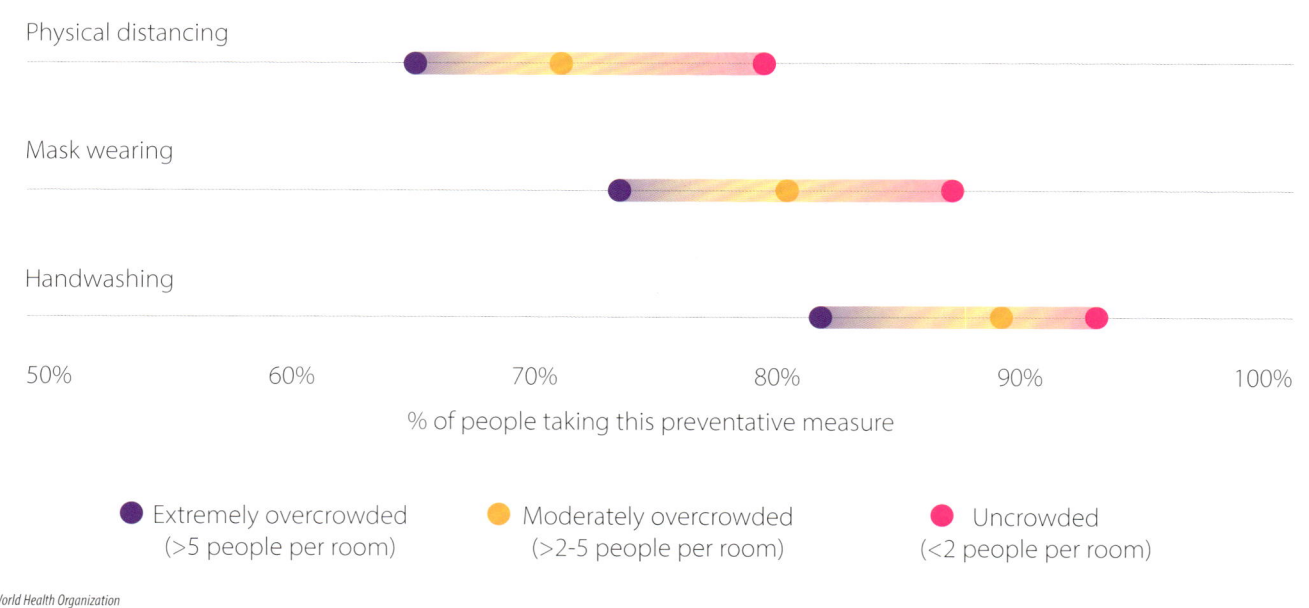

Source: World Health Organization

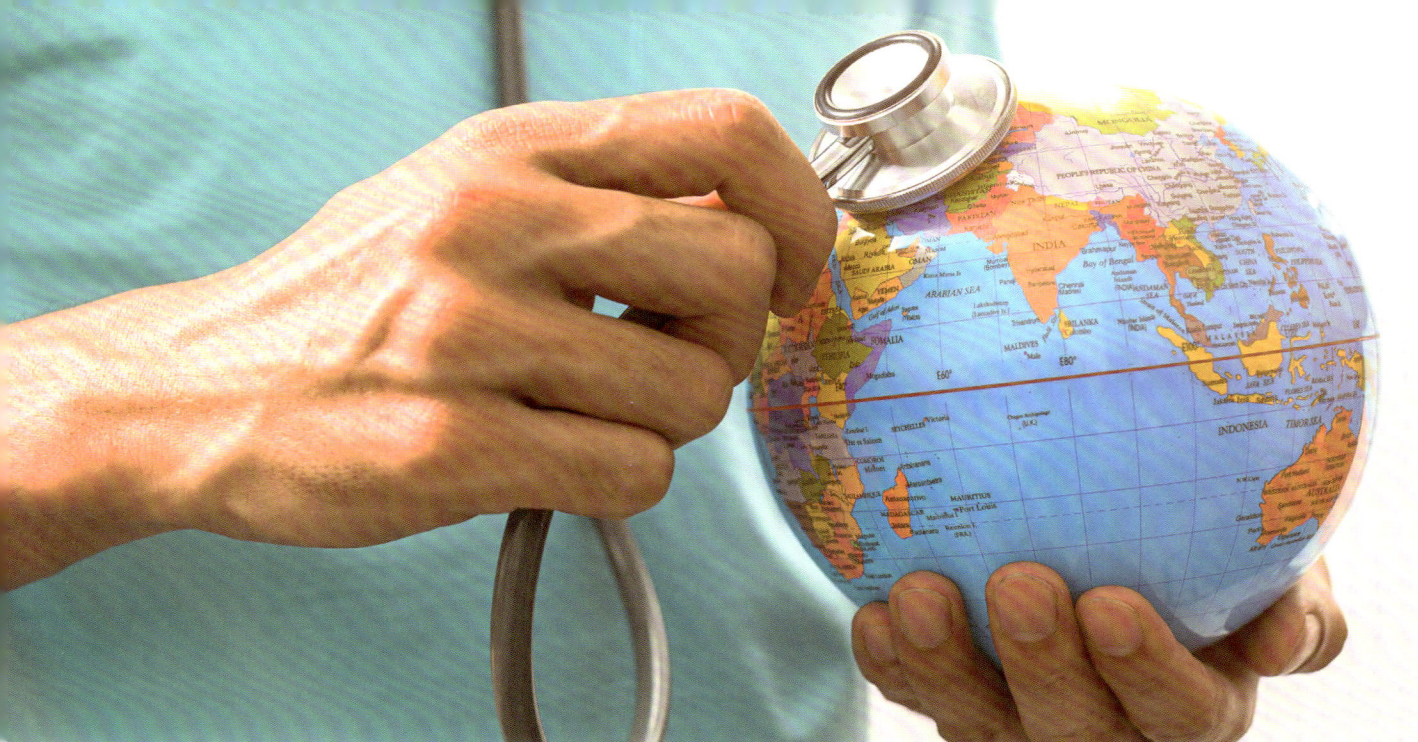

of funding for non-COVID-19 services. The second WHO 'pulse survey' of 135 countries in March 2021 highlighted persistent disruptions at a considerable scale over one year into the pandemic, with 90% of countries reporting one or more disruptions to essential health services.

'All countries must have the necessary capacity and resources to accurately collect and use health data even in the midst of an ongoing crisis', says Dr Tedros Adhanom Ghebreyesus, Director-General of the World Health Organization. 'The COVID-19 pandemic has shown the importance of data and science to build back more resilient health systems and equitably accelerate towards our shared global goals.'

COVID-19 disproportionately impacts vulnerable populations

COVID-19 has exposed persistent inequalities by income, age, race, sex and geographic location. Despite recent global health gains, across the world people continue to face complex, interconnected threats to their health and well-being rooted in social, economic, political and environmental determinants of health.

The pandemic has also revealed significant gaps in country health information systems. While high-resource settings have faced challenges related to overstretched capacity

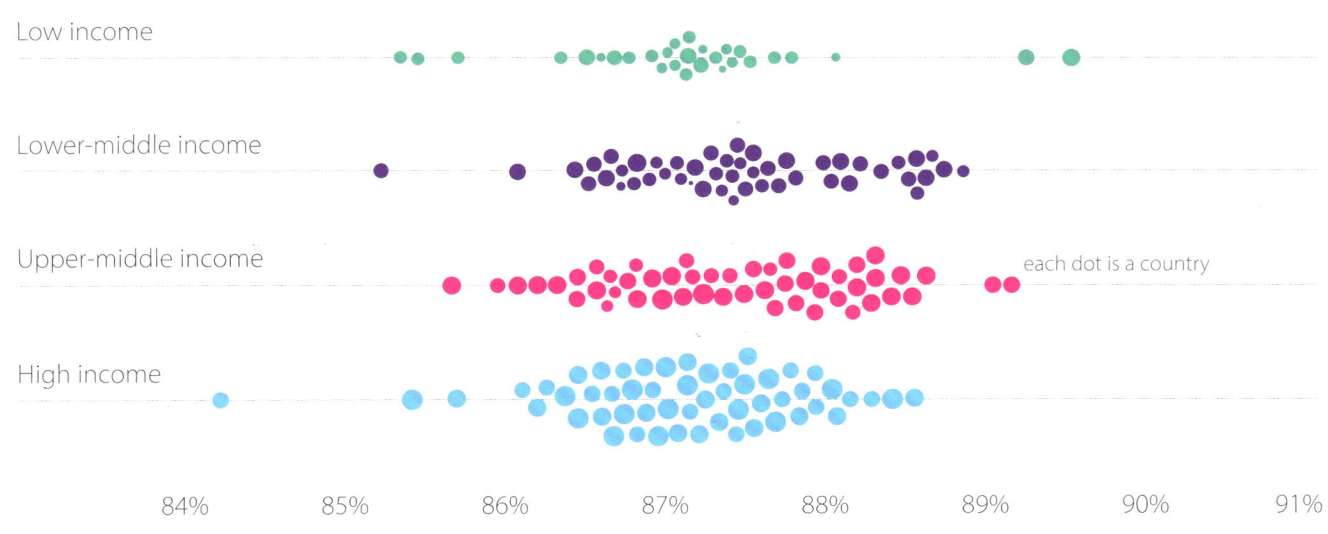

Across the world, where are people living a higher proportion of years in good health?

% of healthy years in life expectancy, 2019

Source: World Health Organization

Global progress and shortfalls towards the Triple Billion targets
2023 targets

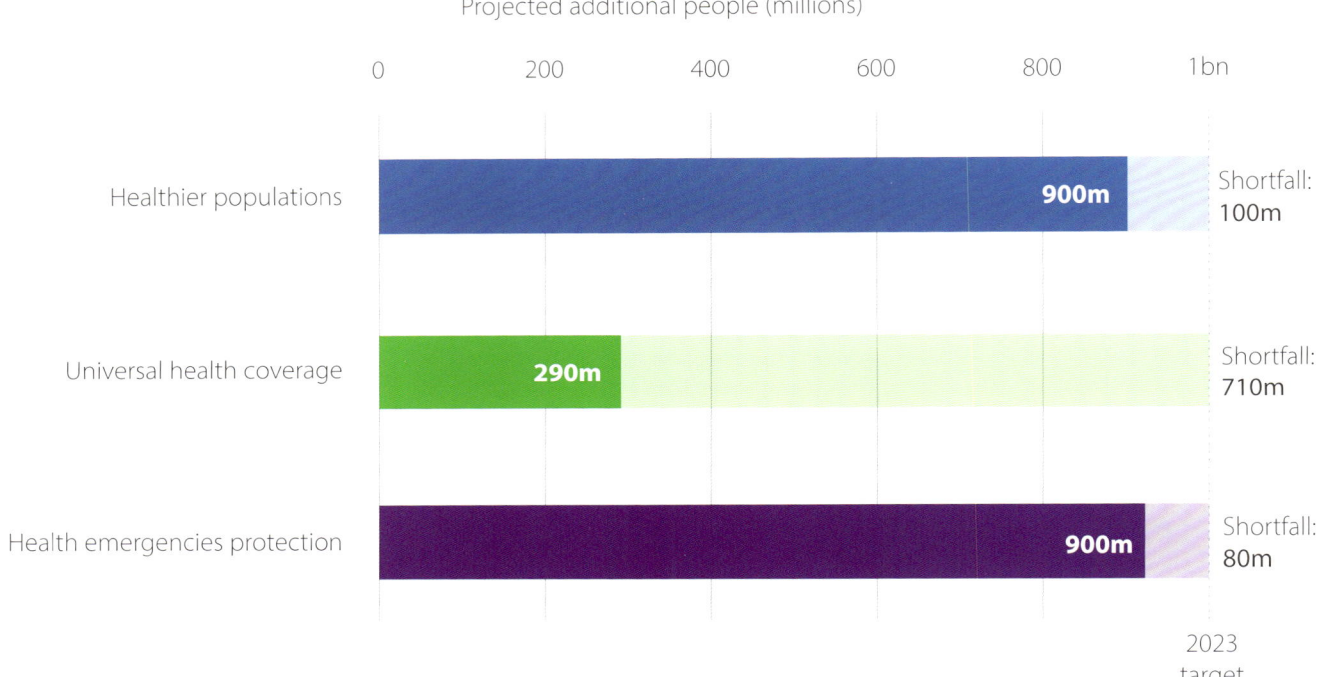

Projected additional people (millions)

- Healthier populations: 900m — Shortfall: 100m
- Universal health coverage: 290m — Shortfall: 710m
- Health emergencies protection: 900m — Shortfall: 80m

Note: analysis does not yet account for impact of COVID-19 on Triple Billion targets

Source: World Health Organization

and fragmentation, weaker health systems risk jeopardizing hard-won health and development gains made in recent decades.

Data from the COVID-19 World Symptoms survey shows a decline in preventive behaviours such as physical distancing, mask wearing and hand washing as household overcrowding increases. Among people living in uncrowded households, 79% reported trying to physically distance themselves compared with 71% in moderately overcrowded and 65% in extremely overcrowded households. Similar trends were observed for hand washing and mask-wearing, underscoring vulnerabilities due to socioeconomic status.

Irrespective of the pandemic, inequalities and data gaps impede targeted interventions. For example, a recent WHO

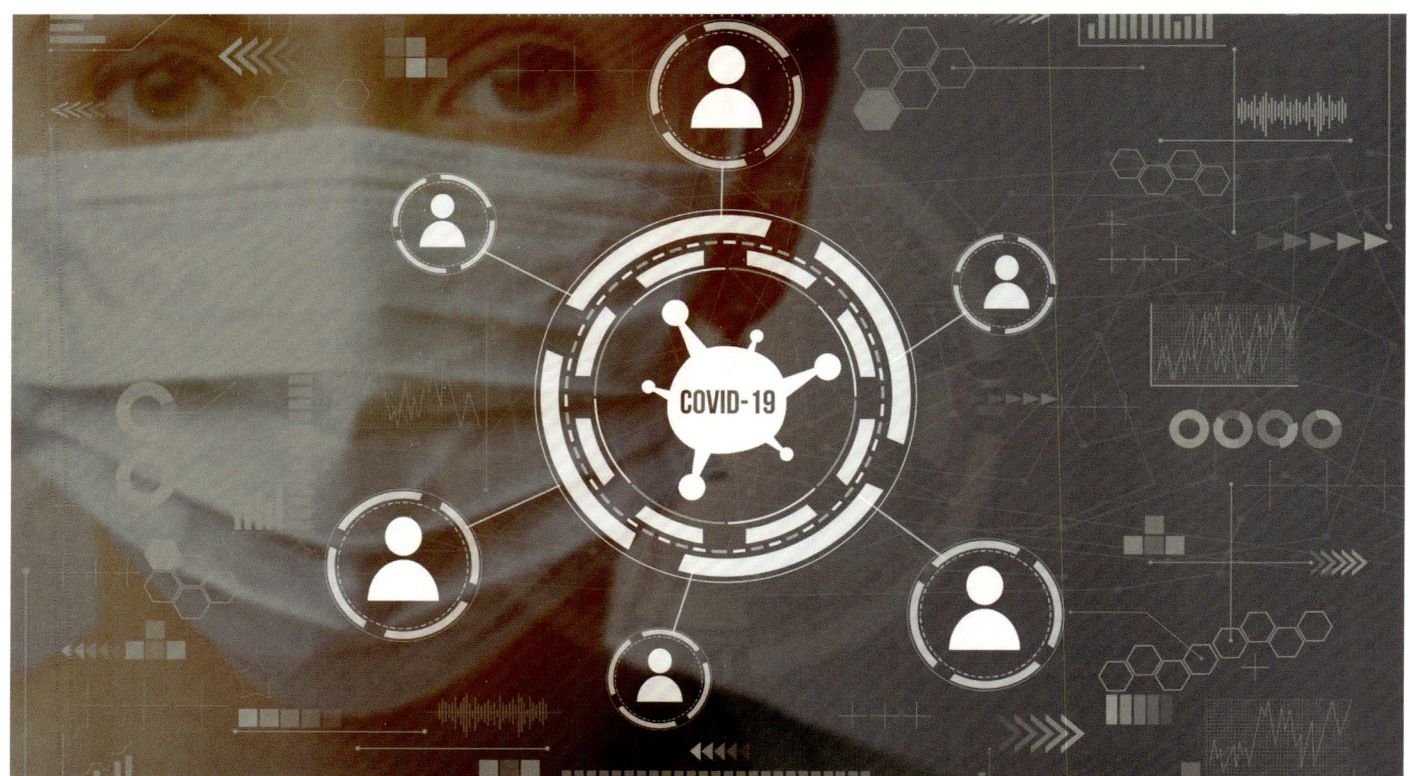

global assessment of health information systems capacity found that only half of countries include disaggregated data in their published national health statistical reports. Investing in strong health information systems is vital to ensure disaggregated data reaches decision-makers and achieve equitable health outcomes.

With stronger, more equitable health information systems we can more accurately measure progress towards the health-related Sustainable Development Goals and WHO's Triple Billion targets. 'We are now less than nine years away from 2030', says Dr Samira Asma, Assistant Director-General for the Division of Data, Analytics and Delivery for Impact at WHO. 'We know where the gaps are, and we have the solutions to address them. What we need now is commitment and investment to accelerate progress and reach our goals.'

Before COVID-19 the world was making progress towards global health goals - but not fast enough

The World Health Statistics 2021 report presents the most up-to-date data and trends on more than 50 health-related indicators for the Sustainable Development Goal and WHO's Triple Billion targets.

The data shows that global life expectancy at birth has increased from 66.8 years in 2000 to 73.3 years in 2019, and healthy life expectancy has increased from 58.3 years to 63.7 years. But even before the pandemic struck, progress was too slow and uneven to meet many targets including reduced premature mortality from noncommunicable diseases, tuberculosis and malaria incidence, and new HIV infections.

'Although we are living extended lives and more years in good health, these are no grounds for complacency', says Dr Bochen Cao, Technical Officer in the Division of Data, Analytics and Delivery for Impact at WHO. 'Many of the underlying health determinants still need critical improvements, and COVID-19 is yet another wake-up call to remind us that our health remains at risk unless urgent actions are taken to close the gaps.'

For instance, while global tobacco use has decreased by 33% since 2000 the prevalence of adult obesity is increasing, and in 2016 up to a quarter of the populations in high-income countries were obese. And although the prevalence of hypertension declined worldwide between 2000 and 2015, it is increasing slightly in low-income countries.

Children and women in low and lower-middle-income countries are also at higher risk of malnutrition including stunting, wasting, and anaemia during pregnancy, while people in upper-middle-income countries are more susceptible to being overweight.

Key Facts

- As of 31 December 2020, COVID-19 had infected over 82 million people and killed more than 1.8 million worldwide.
- Among people living in uncrowded households, 79% reported trying to physically distance themselves compared with 71% in moderately overcrowded and 65% in extremely overcrowded households
- Global tobacco use has decreased by 33% since 2000.
- In 2016 up to a quarter of the populations in high-income countries were obese.
- Global life expectancy at birth has increased from 66.8 years in 2000 to 73.3 years in 2019, and healthy life expectancy has increased from 58.3 years to 63.7 years.

Before COVID-19, many countries were making progress towards universal health coverage. Improvements in the coverage of essential health services were recorded in all income groups and across different types of services, despite persistent inequalities. But financial protection has been deteriorating. As of the latest figures, the proportion of the population spending more than 10% of their household budget on healthcare rose from 9% to 13% between 2000 and 2015, and almost 3% were spending more than 25% of their budget on health care.

Health emergencies protection also requires urgent reform. Despite an increased focus on global health security, COVID-19 has revealed a critical need for a well-coordinated, multisectoral health emergency surge capacity and preparedness at all levels and within all countries. Continuing efforts are needed to improve and maintain early warning systems to mitigate and manage public health risks within the national context and to consider the worldwide pandemic contexts for national health emergency and operational preparedness planning.

20 May 2021

The above information is reprinted with kind permission from the World Health Organization.
© 2023 WHO

www.who.int

What to know about coronaviruses

Coronaviruses cause a range of illnesses, including COVID-19. They typically affect the respiratory tract, but their effects can extend well beyond the respiratory system.

Medically reviewed by Joseph Vinetz, MD — By Adam Felman

At the end of 2019, scientists identified a coronavirus outbreak in China. Experts named the newly identified virus severe acute respiratory syndrome coronavirus 2 (SARS-CoV-2) and the illness that it causes coronavirus disease 19 (COVID-19).

There are many types of coronavirus. Some cause mild illnesses, such as the common cold. Others can cause severe acute respiratory syndrome (SARS) or Middle East respiratory syndrome (MERS), which can be life threatening.

Many coronaviruses are present in animals but do not affect humans. Sometimes, however, a virus mutates in a way that allows it to infect humans. Scientists call these human coronaviruses, or 'HCoVs.'

This article looks at a few coronaviruses that can infect humans, the illnesses they cause, and how they transmit. Specifically, we focus on three dangerous diseases caused by coronaviruses: COVID-19, SARS, and MERS.

What is a coronavirus?

Researchers first identified a coronavirus in 1937. They isolated one that was responsible for a type of bronchitis in birds and had the potential to devastate poultry stocks.

Scientists found evidence of human coronaviruses in the 1960s, in the noses of people with the common cold. Several human coronaviruses cause mild illnesses, including colds.

The name 'coronavirus' refers to the crown-like projections on the pathogen's surface. 'Corona' in Latin means 'halo' or 'crown.'

In humans, coronavirus infections most often occur in the winter and early spring, but they can happen at any time.

COVID-19

Late in 2019, scientists started monitoring the outbreak of a new coronavirus, SARS-CoV-2, which causes COVID-19. They first identified the virus in Wuhan, China.

The virus spread rapidly around the world, and the World Health Organization (WHO) declared a pandemic in March 2020.

The new coronavirus has been responsible for millions of infections globally, and it has caused more than 2 million deaths. The mortality rate varies from country to country. In the United States, it is around 1.7%.

Many researchers believe SARS-CoV-2 first infected bats before spreading to other animals, including humans. Some of the first people with COVID-19 had links to a live animal and seafood market. Overall, however, there is little conclusive information about the origins of the virus. Scientists are still investigating its source and initial pattern of spreading.

Many people with COVID-19 experience a relatively mild form of the disease that does not require specialist treatment. Others develop severe breathing problems and need to spend time in the hospital. In some cases, it is fatal.

Some people who do not have severe symptoms initially go on to develop health issues that continue for weeks or months, according to the Centers for Disease Control and Prevention (CDC).

People with a higher risk of severe COVID-19 symptoms include older adults and those with underlying medical conditions, including high blood pressure, heart and lung problems, diabetes, and cancer.

According to the CDC, most children with COVID-19 have mild or no symptoms. Fewer children have developed COVID-19 than adults. That said, infants and children with certain medical conditions may have an increased risk of severe illness and death.

There may also be a higher risk of severe COVID-19 during pregnancy, as well as an increased risk of issues such as preterm birth. However, the role of the virus in these circumstances remains unclear.

Symptoms of COVID-19

People may start to experience COVID-19 symptoms 2–14 days after exposure to SARS-CoV-2.

Symptoms of COVID-19 include:

- a fever
- chills
- a cough
- shortness of breath or difficulty breathing
- a sore throat
- congestion or a runny nose
- fatigue
- a headache
- muscle pain
- a new loss of taste or smell
- nausea, vomiting, or both
- diarrhoea

Tests can detect the infection, even if there are no symptoms.

As the virus progresses, severe complications can arise. COVID-19 can affect a wide range of body systems and lead to multiple organ failure.

Systemic inequalities in healthcare have increased the risk of illness and death for people in marginalised racial and ethnic groups.

SARS

SARS is a disease caused by an infection with a different coronavirus — SARS-CoV. It can lead to a life threatening form of pneumonia.

SARS first appeared in Asia in February 2003 . The virus then spread to more than two dozen countries, resulting in 8,098 infections and 774 deaths. The last reported cases in humans occurred in a laboratory-related outbreak in China in 2004.

Symptoms of SARS

Early symptoms are flu-like and include :

- a high fever
- a headache
- body aches
- a feeling of discomfort
- mild respiratory symptoms, in some cases

The infection affects both the upper and lower respiratory tracts. After 7–10 days, the person may develop a dry cough. Also, pneumonia, a severe lung infection, often develops.

As SARS progresses, it can lead to failure of the lungs, liver, or heart.

During the outbreak, complications were more common among older adults. According to one source, more than half of those who died from the disease were over the age of 65.

MERS

MERS is a severe respiratory illness caused by the MERS-CoV coronavirus. Scientists first recognized it in 2012 after reports in Saudi Arabia. After that, it spread to other countries, including the U.S.

MERS has not become widespread in the same way as COVID-19. According to reported figures, about 30–40% of people with MERS die from the disease.

Symptoms of MERS

These symptoms include :

- a fever
- breathlessness
- coughing
- nausea, diarrhoea, and vomiting, in some cases

Complications include pneumonia and kidney failure.

The illness spreads through close contact with people who have the infection.

People aged 1–99 years have had MERS, and severe symptoms were more common among older people and those with underlying health conditions or weakened immune systems.

Transmission

Coronavirus infections are contagious, and some of these viruses, including the one that causes COVID-19, spread easily between people. Researchers believe that the viruses transmit via fluids from the respiratory system.

Transmission may happen when a person:

- coughs or sneezes without covering their mouth, dispersing droplets containing the virus into the air
- has physical contact with someone who has the infection
- touches a surface that contains the virus, then touches their nose, eyes, or mouth

Ways of preventing transmission include:

- wearing a face covering in public
- avoiding touching the face, especially the mouth and nose
- always coughing or sneezing into a tissue, then disposing of it and washing the hands right away
- regularly and thoroughly washing the hands

During the ongoing COVID-19 pandemic, people should also do the following, even if they are well:

- Stay home whenever possible.
- Avoid contact with others.
- Wear a face covering in public.
- Stay at least 6 feet away from others in public.

Anyone with symptoms of COVID-19 should isolate at home and rest until the symptoms have passed. Contact a doctor for more information, and let them know if the symptoms seem to be worsening.

Vaccines can help prevent infection with SARS-CoV-2

Summary

Coronaviruses are present in humans and other animals, and some types can cause severe illness.

The common cold is one illness that can result from a coronavirus. Others include SARS, MERS, and COVID-19.

Scientists continue to investigate coronaviruses and monitor for new types and outbreaks

31 January 2021

Design

Design a poster to show the ways to reduce transmission of coronaviruses.

Research

Do some research into how many people were affected by the SARS and MERS viruses, and how the infection and death rates compare to COVID-19.

Show your findings in a graph or infographic.

The above information is reprinted with kind permission from Medical News Today.
Republished from What to know about coronaviruses by Adam Felman by permission of Medical News Today.
© 2004-2022 Healthline Media UK Ltd, Brighton, UK, a Red Ventures Company

www.medicalnewstoday.com

The recent monkeypox outbreak is a reminder that our interconnected world has its dangers

These cases show how our modern, mobile, interconnected world, which enables us to travel quickly from continent to continent, does make countries across the globe more vulnerable to occasional imported infections.

By Jimmy Whitworth

The report of two apparently unconnected cases of monkeypox in the UK within one week was a surprise for public health officials. No cases of the virus had been reported previously in the UK, or even more widely in Europe.

The two cases had both travelled to the UK from Nigeria, where they would have contracted their infections. There have been reports of an increase in cases of monkeypox in Nigeria and elsewhere in west Africa in the past few months, and this is likely to explain why we have seen these infections for the first time in the UK.

A third case has now been reported, this time in a healthcare worker who was infected in the UK while caring for one of the imported cases. Public Health England has said that the transmission occurred before the diagnosis was made. This is often a risky period as stringent infection control procedures may not be in place before a diagnosis is made or even suspected. Whether this transmission was bad luck or due to a lapse in basic standard precautions is not clear.

Monkeypox emerged in west and central Africa in the 1980s. It is thought that this is related to stopping routine smallpox vaccination once that disease had been eradicated, leaving the population exposed to the closely related but much milder monkeypox. Over 100 cases of monkeypox were reported in Nigeria in 2017.

The infection is usually contracted from small rodents in the African forest and is not easily transmitted from human to human. It causes a typical acute viral illness with fever, pains and malaise, with a typical rash of pox lesions, as seen in chickenpox or smallpox.

Most cases recover with careful nursing in a few weeks, although it can be fatal in around one to 10 per cent of cases. Why there has been a rise in cases in Nigeria is not clear but increases in rodent populations or more contact with humans are possible reasons.

Public health measures include isolation of cases and strict infection control. If the authorities actively identify the contacts of the cases and can keep them under observation there is very little risk of any sustained transmission in the UK.

Since the cases arrived, contacts have been offered smallpox vaccination which will reduce the risk of transmission still further. It is possible more cases will be identified in travellers to the UK, and health authorities will need to be vigilant and consider the possibility of monkeypox in patients with a consistent medical and travel history.

We of course wish those affected a full, speedy recovery but isolated monkeypox cases pose no great cause for concern in the UK. However these cases are another reminder that our modern, mobile, interconnected world, which enables us to travel quickly from continent to continent, does make countries across the globe more vulnerable to occasional imported infections – many of which are more dangerous to humans than monkeypox.

This year we have seen bigger than normal outbreaks of Lassa fever (Nigeria), Nipah virus (India), and of course the Democratic Republic of Congo, supported by various global organisations, is still tackling its second Ebola virus outbreak of 2018.

The UK's expertise, experience and robust health system means we are well prepared to handle these isolated cases and offer excellent care to those affected. Other countries, however, are not so fortunate.

It's imperative that the UK continues its strong support to help low-income countries stop disease outbreaks in their tracks. This will save lives 'on the ground', and will also help prevent dangerous infections reaching our shores.

Jimmy Whitworth is a professor of international public health at the London School of Hygiene and Tropical Medicine

29 September 2022

The above information is reprinted with kind permission from *The Independent*.
© independent.co.uk 2023

www.independent.co.uk

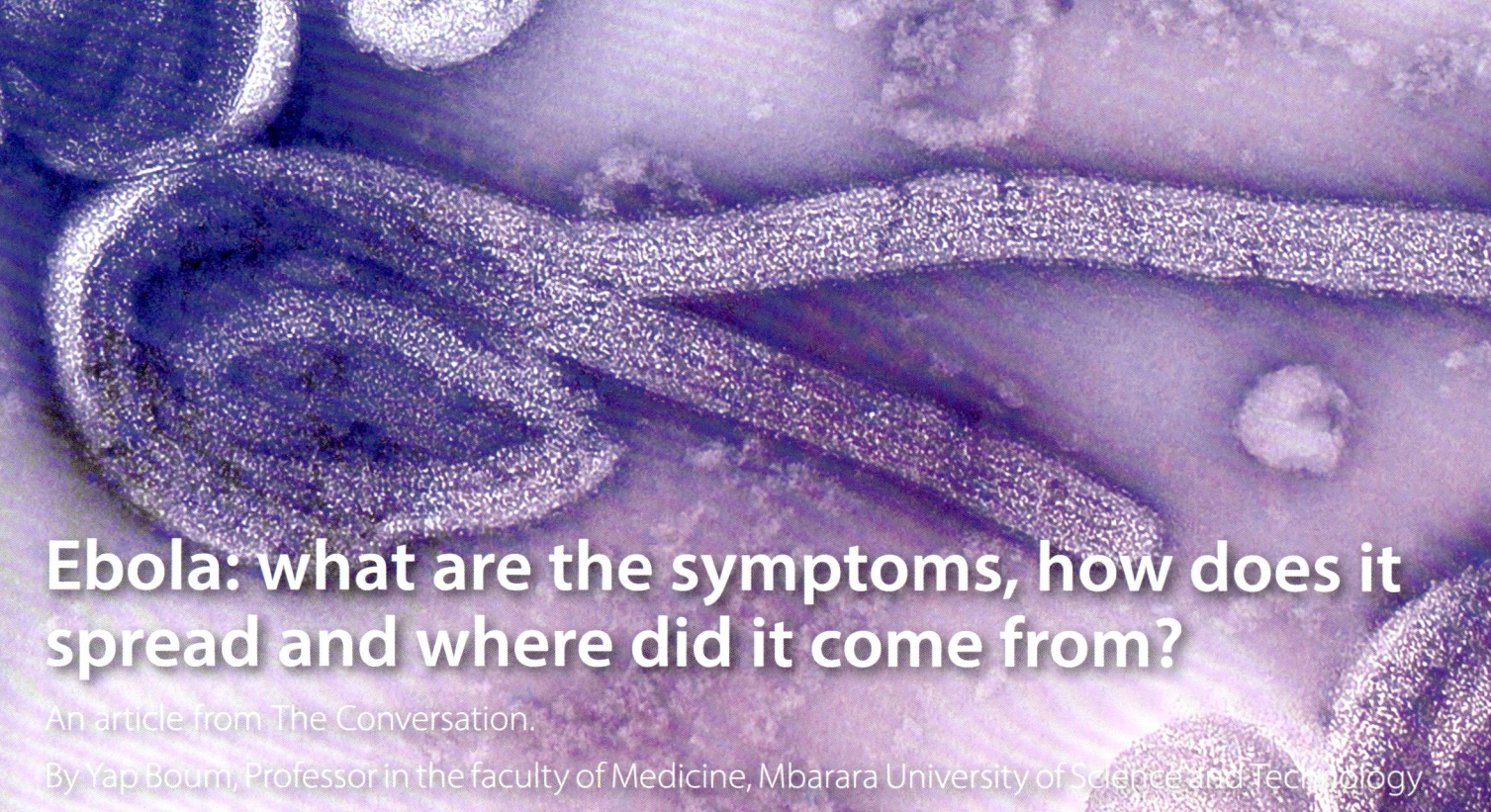

Ebola: what are the symptoms, how does it spread and where did it come from?

An article from The Conversation.

By Yap Boum, Professor in the faculty of Medicine, Mbarara University of Science and Technology

Uganda health authorities have declared an outbreak of Ebola disease. Ebola outbreaks emerge periodically in several African countries, most notably in the Democratic Republic of Congo (DRC). Public health expert Yap Boum, who has been involved in managing Ebola outbreaks in the past, answers some key questions about Ebola's history, treatment, and how to keep safe.

What are the origins of the virus?

Ebola is an old and deadly disease that was discovered in 1976 near the Ebola river in northern DRC. The virus was named after the river. It was discovered by scientists including Jean-Jacques Muyembe – a Congolese microbiologist and general director of the DRC Institut National pour la Recherche Biomedicale – and researchers from the Institute of Tropical Medicine, including Stefaan Pattyn, Guido van der Groen and Peter Piot.

Professor Muyembe was called to the village of Yambuku in northern Zaire (now DRC) where a mysterious illness had broken out. He took a sample and sent it to the Institute of Tropical Medicine laboratory in Belgium, where the virus was isolated.

Since then, there have been five identified Ebola virus strains, four of which are known to cause disease in humans: Ebola virus (Zaire ebolavirus); Sudan virus (Sudan ebolavirus); Taï Forest virus (Taï Forest ebolavirus, formerly Côte d'Ivoire ebolavirus); and Bundibugyo virus (Bundibugyo ebolavirus).

It's a zoonotic disease (animal-borne) though the natural reservoir host of Ebola virus remains unknown. However, bats are the most likely reservoir.

What are the symptoms of Ebola?

While the signs and symptoms may appear between 2 and 21 days after contact with the virus, they usually appear between 8 and 10 days.

They are quite similar to many tropical diseases, especially malaria and typhoid fever, with which they share symptoms such as:

- fever
- aches and pains, such as severe headache and muscle and joint pain
- weakness and fatigue
- sore throat
- loss of appetite
- abdominal pain
- diarrhoea and vomiting
- unexplained haemorrhaging, bleeding or bruising.

The main differences appear in the late stages of infection. These symptoms might include red eyes, skin rash and hiccups.

Can it be treated?

The Ebola virus disease can now be treated. The PALM clinical trial – implemented between 2018 and 2020 in the DRC – has evaluated four drug candidates. Two of them – Inmazeb and Ebanga – were approved by the US Food and Drug Administration in October and December 2020 to treat the Ebola virus disease caused by the Ebola virus. They are made available to patients by the World Health Organization

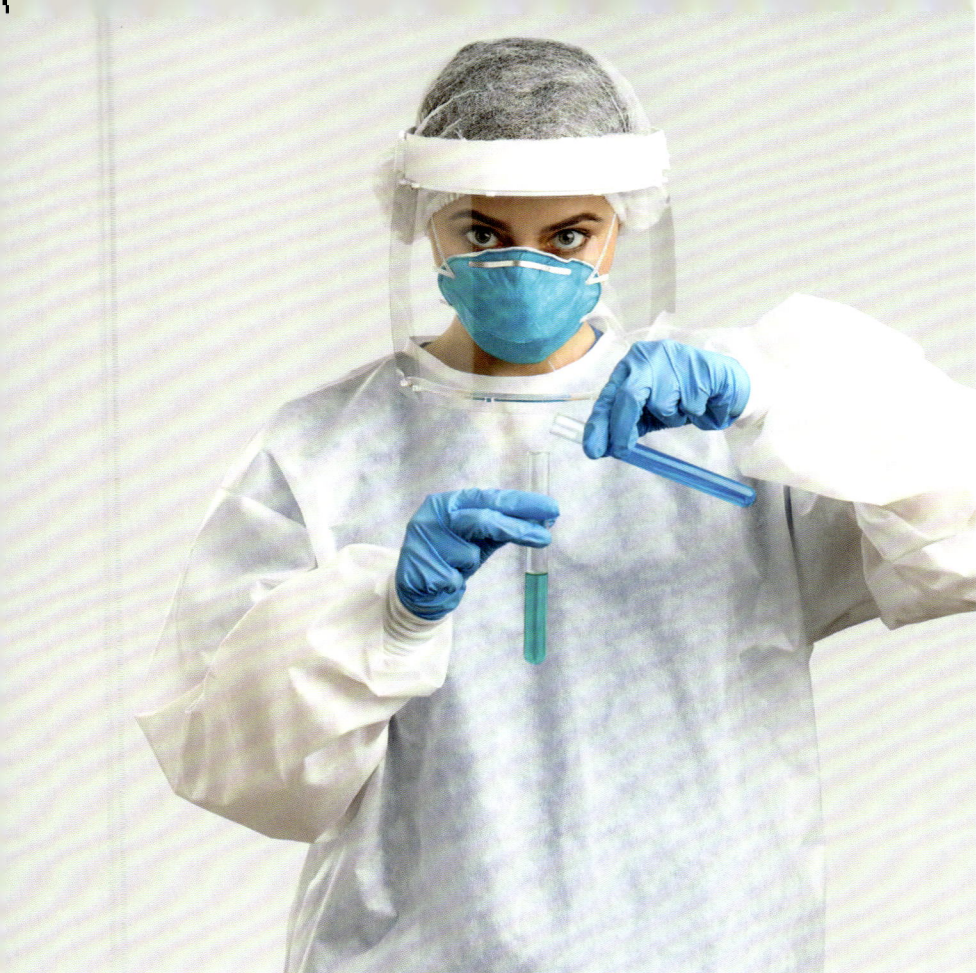

(WHO) during Ebola outbreaks and aren't available in the market.

Inmazeb is a combination of three monoclonal antibodies and Ebanga is a single monoclonal antibody. Monoclonal antibodies (often abbreviated as mAbs) are proteins produced in a lab or other manufacturing facility that act like natural antibodies to stop a germ such as a virus from replicating after it has infected a person.

Ebanga was isolated from a human survivor of the 1995 Ebola outbreak in Kikwit in the DRC who maintained circulating antibodies against the Ebola virus for more than a decade after infection.

Without treatment the average case fatality rate is approximately 50%. But it has ranged from 25% to 90% in past outbreaks.

Can it be prevented?

People can be vaccinated against one strain, the Zaire Ebola virus. It became a preventable disease following the validation of one vaccine candidate during the Ca Suffit Ebola clinical trial in 2015 in Guinea. The Ebola vaccine rVSV-ZEBOV (called Ervebo®) was approved by the US Food and Drug Administration in December 2019. This vaccine is given as a single dose vaccine and has been found to be safe and protective with a reported 100% efficacy.

Though it has not yet been approved by the US Food and Drug Administration, Johnson & Johnson has a two-dose vaccine for the Zaire strain that was used under emergency use in 2019 during an Ebola outbreak in the DRC. This vaccine requires an initial dose and a 'booster' dose 56 days later and could be made available through the WHO during outbreaks.

How can you protect yourself?

Ebola is a highly transmissible disease but, aside from vaccination for the Zaire strain, its spread can be prevented through behavioural measures.

People should avoid contact with blood and body fluids – such as urine, faeces, saliva, sweat, vomit, breast milk, amniotic fluid, semen and vaginal fluids – of people who are sick. People should also avoid contact with their personal items which might have traces of these fluids.

People who were previously infected can still carry the disease in their semen.

Because it's a zoonotic disease – that is, transmitted from animal to humans – people should avoid contact with bats, forest antelopes, nonhuman primates (such as monkeys and chimpanzees) and wild meat and blood especially in endemic areas.

Lastly, funeral or burial practices that involve touching the body of someone who may have died from Ebola should be avoided. Experience in West Africa shows these burial practices to be among the super spreaders of the Ebola virus.

Ebola virus disease is a deadly disease that is preventable and curable. The next step is the local production of diagnostics, vaccines and drugs to ensure that endemic countries control their own stock and can make them available to their population. Africa can't be left behind once more when it comes to diagnostics, vaccines and treatment, as it has been during the COVID pandemic and monkeypox outbreaks.

30 September 2022

THE CONVERSATION

The above information is reprinted with kind permission from The Conversation.
© 2010-2023, The Conversation Trust (UK) Limited

www.theconversation.com

Ebola outbreak re-ignites debate over international travel checks in UK and US

The US imposes checks on arrivals from Uganda – but will it help halt the potential spread of disease?

By Will Brown, Africa correspondent, in Nairobi

The debate about the value of travel checks and restrictions has reemerged after a strain of Ebola with no known vaccine reached the Ugandan capital – with the US and UK diverging in their response.

Since the hemorrhagic virus was detected in mid-September, roughly 30 deaths and 60 confirmed cases have been detected across the east African county.

While the vast majority have been in relatively rural areas in the centre of Uganda, fears were raised this week after officials announced a man had died in Kampala. On Thursday it was confirmed that the man's wife, who had just given birth, had also been infected.

The capital is an international city home to about three million people, with sprawling slums where the virus could spread rapidly.

While there are no direct flights to the UK, there are routes from Kampala straight to Amsterdam, Brussels and regional travel hubs including Addis Ababa, Istanbul and Doha.

Last week, the US imposed travel checks on all passengers arriving from Uganda. Travellers who have visited the east African country within the previous 21 days must pass through New York-JFK, Newark, Atlanta, Chicago O'Hare or Washington Dulles airports to be checked.

But there is significant debate about whether such moves actually help halt the potential spread of disease.

'[The] screening of travellers returning from Uganda is not an effective control measure,' the European Centre for Disease Control said in a statement. The agency suggested it had seen no benefit in imposing checks on incoming passengers during the massive outbreak of Ebola from 2014 – 2016 in west Africa.

'Screening incoming travellers is time and resource-consuming and will not identify effectively infected cases,' the ECDC added.

Others, though, say limited and proportional health checks are an important tool.

'If this disease is going to travel around the world, it will go through airports,' Prof Devi Sridhar, chair of global public health at the University of Edinburgh, told the *Telegraph*.

'I think what the US did is quite smart. This is not restrictions. This is not a ban. This is not Covid-19. This is checking and getting more information so that if any symptoms develop, we can catch the infection fast and respond,' she said.

Prof Sridhar added that it is unlikely that anyone with visible symptoms would board a plane as 'you definitely would not be well enough', but you may be within the 21-

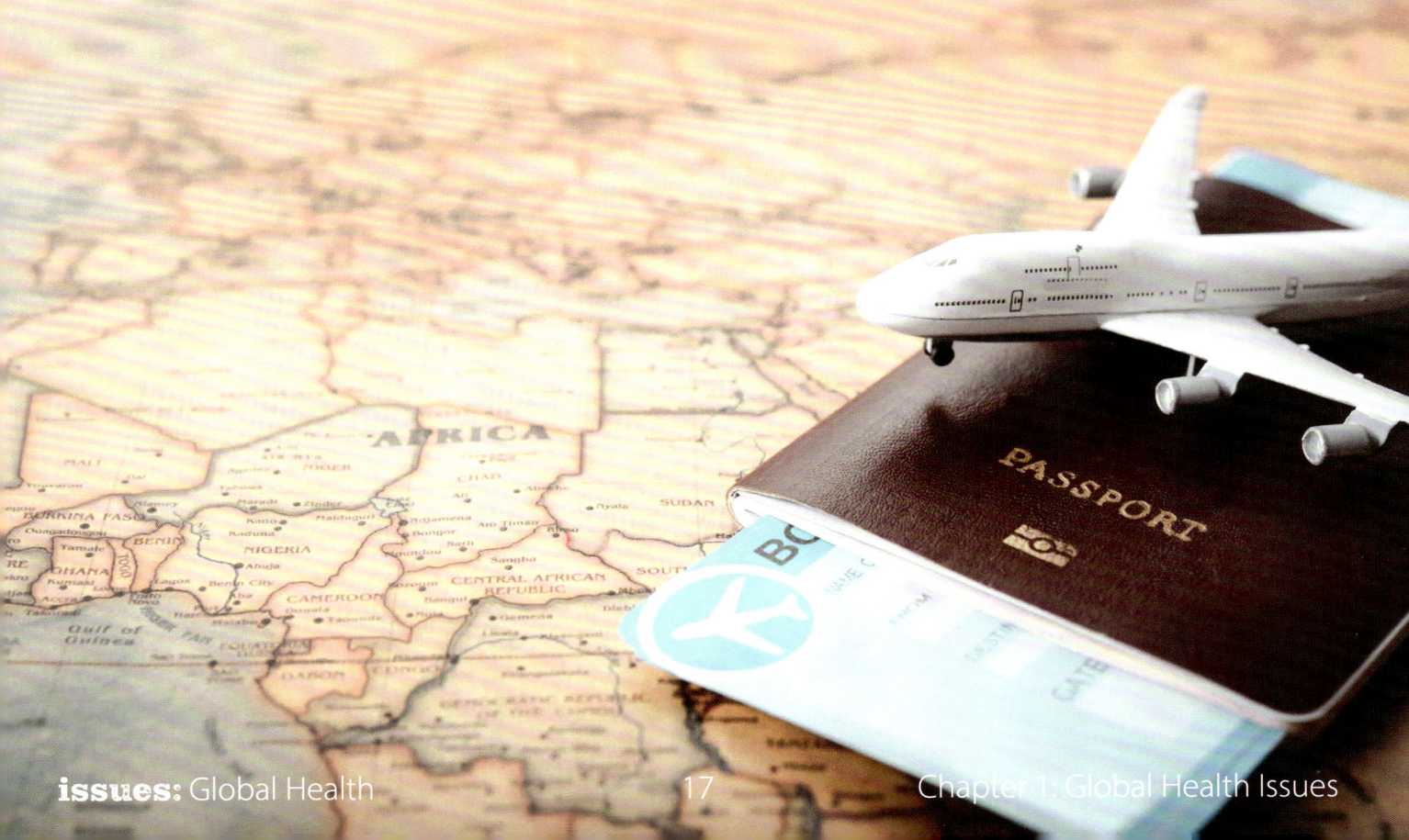

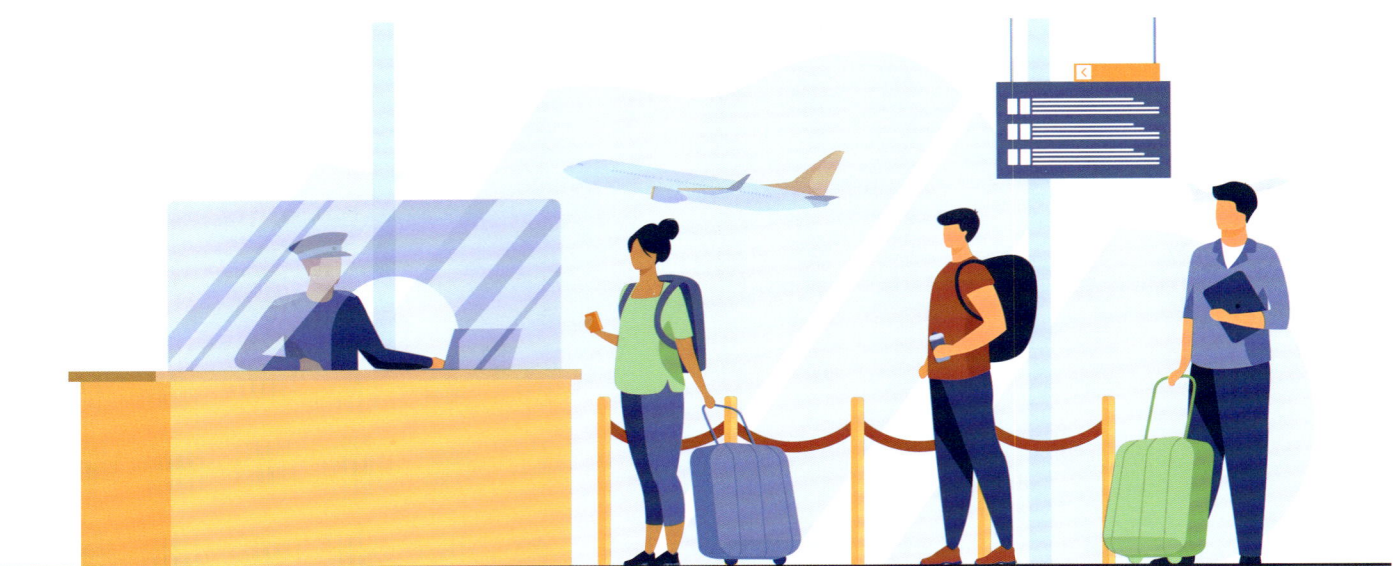

day incubation period, meaning you could still develop symptoms in due course.

As well as having their temperatures and 'visible symptoms' checked on arrival in America, travellers will be asked for contact details and given information about where to go should they develop a fever. The US government has reportedly also asked for the names of contact cases to bar them from flights.

Yet many say checks are more targeted and appropriate if applied to people leaving Uganda, rather than arriving elsewhere. This is already happening – heat detectors have been deployed at Entebbe airport in Kampala.

For now, there are few signs that Britain is about to follow America's lead, and the UK Health Security agency has insisted the risk to Britain remains 'very low'.

Symptom vigilance

The UKHSA told doctors to be 'vigilant to the symptoms', especially in those who have recently returned from Uganda, and ensure they have adequate stocks of PPE. It has also activated the returning workers scheme, which ensures people who come back from Uganda have a point of contact if they start to feel unwell.

Debates around travel checks echo conversations during the coronavirus pandemic. Although the two diseases are very different, the World Health Organization was criticised for not advocating for travel bans soon enough given the way Covid-19 spreads.

The WHO, which is wary of offending its members, is often concerned that these measures would hinder transparency and create incentives not to share data.

But UK experts involved in the response told the Telegraph restrictions that may help curb Covid would not necessarily work for Ebola. The key strategy is to closely monitor those considered high risk – such as health workers helping on the frontlines – as they are most likely to bring the virus to Britain.

Professor Richard Sullivan, co-director of the Conflict and Health Research Group at King's College London, added that the UK is already capable of tracking people coming in from Uganda and any measures must remain 'sensible and proportional'.

'There are a lot of lessons which have been learned from dealing with Ebola in first West Africa and then in Eastern Congo,' he said.

'The UKHSA has a lot more intelligence than it used to and its processes and methodologies are a lot better than they were prior to Covid. It can utilise assets from both civilian and military sectors. That helps to bridge the gaps. Both of those sides bring very distinct expertise.'

He added that the UK should remain cautious and new measures may be needed in due course, but for now Britain's response has been appropriate.

'If you overreact, you desensitise populations,' Prof Sullivan said. 'You need [to be] very careful. You can't throw the kitchen sink at it every time. We've seen this in Eastern Congo and Uganda before – you see these spikes, and then the government gets on top of it very quickly.'

The world has battled sporadic Ebola outbreaks since 1976, the most deadly of which killed more than 11,000 people across Sierra Leone, Guinea and Liberia between 2014 and 2016.

While a vaccine has been developed for the standard Ebola-Zaire variant, the strain spreading in Uganda is the Ebola-Sudanese variant, which has no known shot.

World Health Organization chief Tedros Adhanom Ghebreyesus said on Wednesday that clinical trials would start within weeks on vaccines to combat the Sudan strain – including a candidate created by scientists at the University of Oxford.

14 October 2022

The above information is reprinted with kind permission from *The Telegraph*.
© Telegraph Media Group Limited 2022

www.telegraph.co.uk

World Malaria Report 2021 – A more accurate picture of the malaria burden in Africa

By Professor Tom Churcher

Today, the World Health Organisation (WHO) published its annual *World Malaria Report*. The report shines a new light on the burden of malaria, using updated methodology to calculate the number of malaria deaths among children under five years of age. This new statistical method provides a much more precise cause-of-death estimate for young children for all diseases, including malaria, and is now being applied across the WHO.

The findings of the *2021 World Malaria Report* are stark, revealing that malaria leads to more total deaths than previously thought: 627,000 in 2020, a significant increase from the 409,000 deaths reported in 2019. This increase is due in part to the revised number of malaria deaths among children under the age of five, with malaria now accounting for 7.8% of deaths, an increase from the previous 4.8%. The higher numbers also reflect wider issues with malaria control, as advances have stalled in recent years and there has been considerable disruption caused by the COVID-19 pandemic.

The new report also underscores that Africa shoulders an even heavier burden of malaria than previously accounted for, with 96% of global deaths from the disease occurring in the African region this past year.

The updated methodology is outlined in an article published in *The Lancet*. This highlights that a broad understanding of the causes of mortality among the under-five age group is essential to identify appropriate targets and interventions to address mortality in young children. Many countries do not have functioning vital registration systems to directly report underlying causes of death. The new methodology overcomes this by using more diverse primary input data – such as verbal autopsy – to generate more reliable estimates.

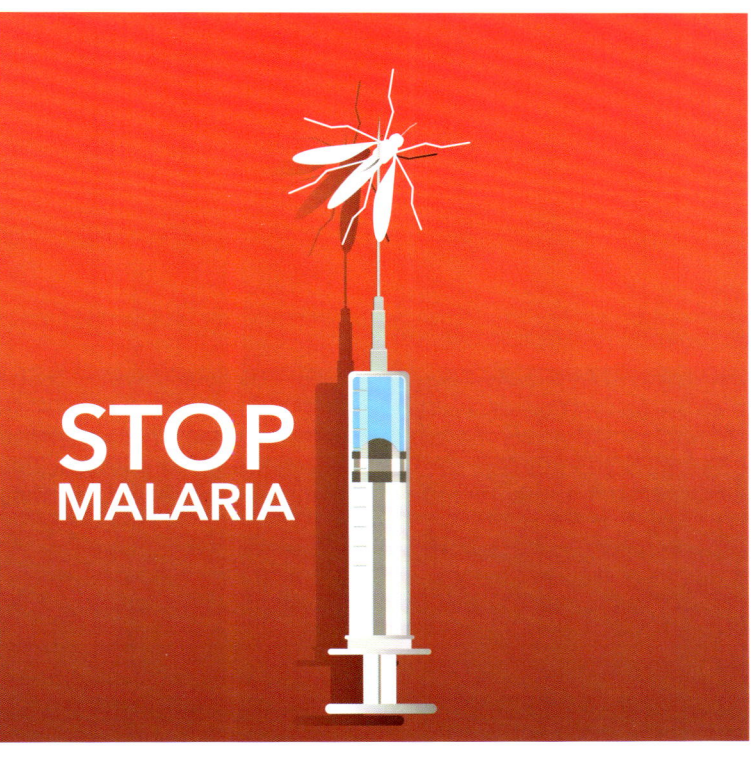

Accurate data plays a critical role in assessing the impact of malaria, planning interventions and placing malaria at the forefront of the global health agenda. There are real challenges associated with data collection and forecasting, worsened by existing data gaps – for example, only eight African countries out of 54 have a compulsory system to register deaths. In light of this, it is imperative that the methodologies we use in research come as close as possible to providing an accurate picture of the malaria burden.

Going forward, the updated methodology will help provide a more reliable picture of the malaria burden in Africa. Good data to base decisions on is essential to indicate where more investment and research are needed to reduce preventable deaths and improve health outcomes. Our work at Imperial College London is investigating how limited malaria budgets can be best used to reduce the burden of disease. Much can be done with existing tools though new technology and innovations are urgently needed.

We have known how to control malaria for over a century. It shows the neglect of investment in the health of communities suffering from the disease that we are only now understanding how great a toll it causes. It is essential that we take this information to galvanise funding and redouble our efforts to tackle malaria world-wide, saving lives.

6 December 2021

Key Facts

- 96% of deaths from malaria occurred in Africa.
- 2020 saw an increase to 627,000 deaths from malaria, 218,000 more than in 2019.
- 7.8% of deaths were children under 5-years-old.

The above information is reprinted with kind permission from Target Malaria.
© Target Malaria 2023

www.targetmalaria.org

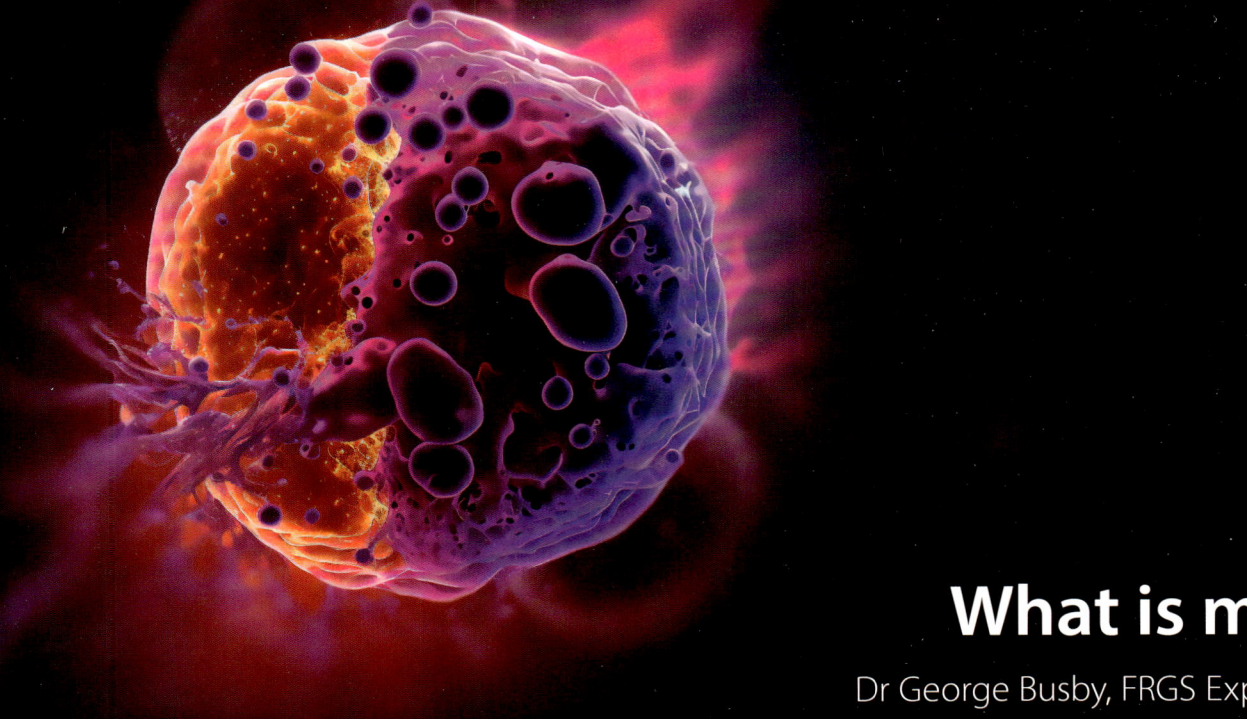

What is malaria?

Dr George Busby, FRGS Expedition Leader

Malaria is a globally important parasitic infectious disease transmitted between humans by mosquitoes.

In 2016, 216 million people worldwide were infected and over 400,000 people died from malaria, around 90% of whom were in sub-Saharan Africa; that's one death every two minutes. This is a tragedy for a disease which is largely treatable.

Eliminating malaria is an international priority which doesn't just save lives but contributes to key global Sustainable Development Goals.

The challenge of controlling malaria

Malaria is transmitted between humans by mosquitoes. Although there are five species of malaria that infect humans, most human disease is caused by just two, Plasmodium vivax and P. falciparum. Together they account for over 400,000 deaths every year, ninety per cent of which occur in Africa.

Significant international effort over the last 20 years means that this number is now around half of what it was in the year 2000. Although malaria transmission is influenced by a number of factors, including climate and land use, it is likely that the main contributors to recent reductions in transmission have been human interventions: the widespread use of insecticide treated bednets, which stop infected mosquitoes from biting people and therefore infecting them, and the better use of drugs to treat disease. It is with renewed confidence then, that the global community has articulated a grand plan to eradicate malaria by 2040.

However, there are at least two important sets of challenges to this ambitious proposal. Firstly, the fight against malaria is being prolonged by a lack of sustained financial and political commitment and regional collaboration at the highest levels.

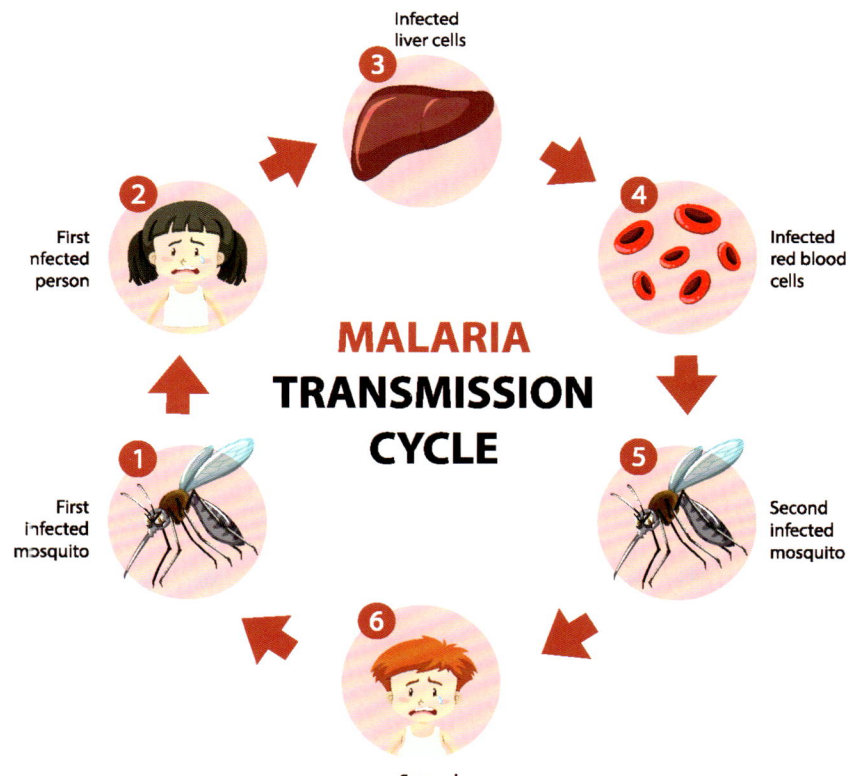

Recent progress is fragile and dependent upon continued funding into the generation and application of interventions at scale. The last thing that the global fight against malaria needs now is complacency lest it become a victim of its own recent, yet historically modest, success.

The second set of challenges relate to the biology of malaria. Just as we are starting to make real gains, the parasite is beginning to fight back, and progress is in danger of being reversed because the parasite is evolving resistance to our drugs and this resistance is spreading. Therefore a crucial part of the global strategy for malaria control is to monitor the spread of antimalarial drug resistance, and identify and contain drug resistant strains when they're found.

On top of this, the dynamics of malaria transmission are complex. For example, as parasite prevalence drops, fewer people are infected, which is clearly a good thing. However, this reduction in malaria endemicity (disease intensity) alters the rules of engagement between people and parasite. In the most endemic settings, many people will be infected by parasites, leading to high levels of asymptomatic infection due to the acquisition of functional immunity that comes from frequent exposure to the parasite. But as endemicity drops, by definition the number of people infected drops which leads to lower levels of natural immunity. Both the spread of drug-resistant infections in endemic regions, and the dynamics of infection in low endemicity settings, can therefore behave more like a disease outbreak.

The case for surveillance

So, to control and eventually eliminate malaria we need to continue to push for financial and political action and develop innovative ways of monitoring parasite and mosquito populations. We need to be able to assess levels of antimalarial drug and insecticide resistance, to understand where resistance first occurs and how it spreads, and to

SYMPTOMS OF MALARIA

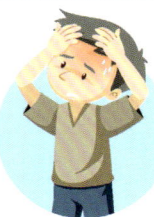
Headache
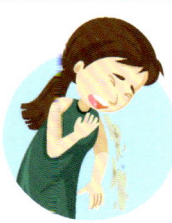
Vomiting
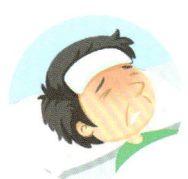
Fever
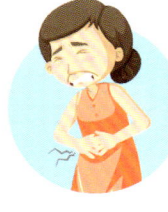
Nausea
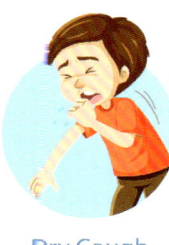
Dry Cough

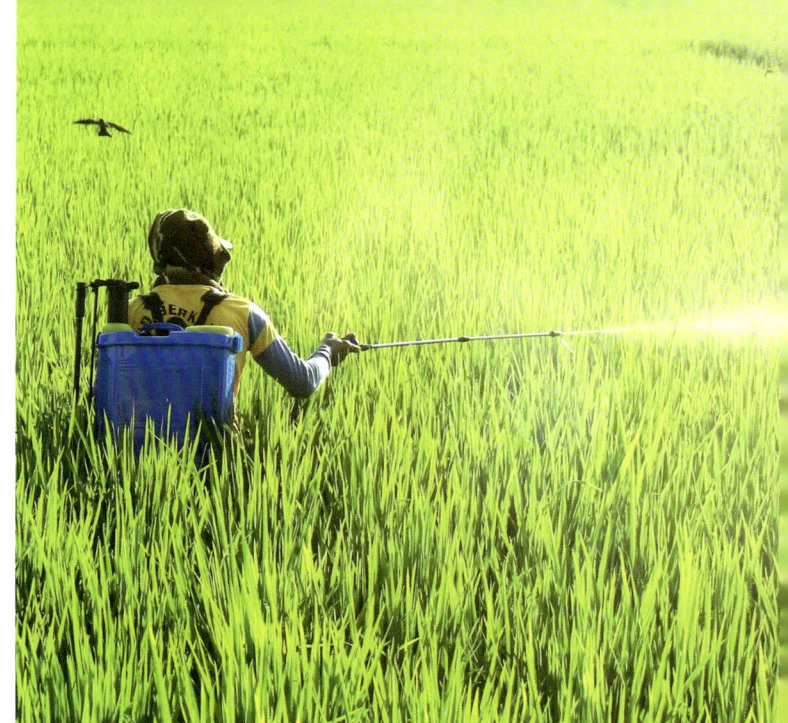

Key Facts

- In 2016, 216 million people worldwide were infected and over 400,000 people died from malaria.
- One person every two minutes dies from malaria.
- 90% of deaths from malaria happen in Africa.
- In just twenty years, deaths from malaria have halved.

identify how interventions are affecting populations. What we need, in other words, is some sort of surveillance system.

A number of different types of data are currently used to understand malaria parasite and vector populations, but none has more potential for inferring key aspects of populations than genomic analysis. DNA sequencing can provide both up-to-date information about which drugs a parasite is resistant to and where a new infection comes from. This is because drug resistance is the result of mutations in the parasite genome, and by comparing an unknown parasite genome to a reference database, we can understand where it comes from.

Traditionally, genome sequencing has been expensive and lab-based, and global parasite reference datasets have been unavailable. However, recent advances in mobile genetic sequencing and the development of cloud-based genome analytics with MalariaGEN, the largest repository of parasite and mosquito sequence data in the world, mean that we now have the tools to take genetic sequencing into the field and provide the necessary information to malaria control programs, in close to real time.

The above information is reprinted with kind permission from Mobile Malaria Project.
© Mobile Malaria Project 2023

www.mobilemalaria.com

New malaria vaccine comes a step closer as experts say it's 'the best yet'

Latest trials on the R21 delight its creators who hope it can be approved next year but comes with fears that UK is set to cut the global health investment that helped make it possible.

By Lizzie Davies

The co-inventor of a vaccine that could eradicate malaria has said he hopes it could be approved by as early as next year after the latest trial results were successful.

Professor Adrian Hill, co-creator of the AstraZeneca Covid vaccine, said it was 'the best [malaria] vaccine yet'. He has previously said he believes R21 could help to reduce deaths from the disease by 70% by 2030 and eradicate it by 2040.

But speaking as the success of the R21 vaccine tests were revealed, Hill, director of Oxford University's Jenner Institute, said it would be tragic if Britain cut funding just as scientists were poised to make 'a real impact' against malaria. He has implored the new British prime minister Liz Truss not to squander cutting-edge UK innovation by 'turning off the taps' on global health funding.

Results from testing in Burkina Faso showed that R21 – already shown to be 77% effective after the initial doses – maintains its high efficacy after a single booster jab.

Researchers hope that the vaccine could be approved by the World Health Organization next year, assuming a larger ongoing trial throws up no unexpected problems.

But Hill also cautioned that getting the vaccine into the arms of tens of millions of African children who most need it would be a challenge without funding.

The body that provides more than half of all financing for the world's malaria programmes, the Global Fund to Fight Aids, Tuberculosis and Malaria, has warned that unless it receives significantly more money from leading donor countries such as the UK at its pledging conference this month, it will not be able to get the fight against those diseases back on track after the Covid pandemic.

The UK has not yet said what it will pledge in New York, but the fund is thought to have asked for about £1.8 billion. As foreign secretary, Truss outlined a strategy for overseas aid marked by an overall spending reduction and a retreat from the funding of multilateral organisations like the Global Fund.

'It's incredibly important that the Global Fund is properly refunded. What they do is absolutely amazing,' said Hill. 'I hope the new prime minister will be very keen to recognise the importance of doing what the UK [the fund's third-biggest donor] has done so well in the past.'

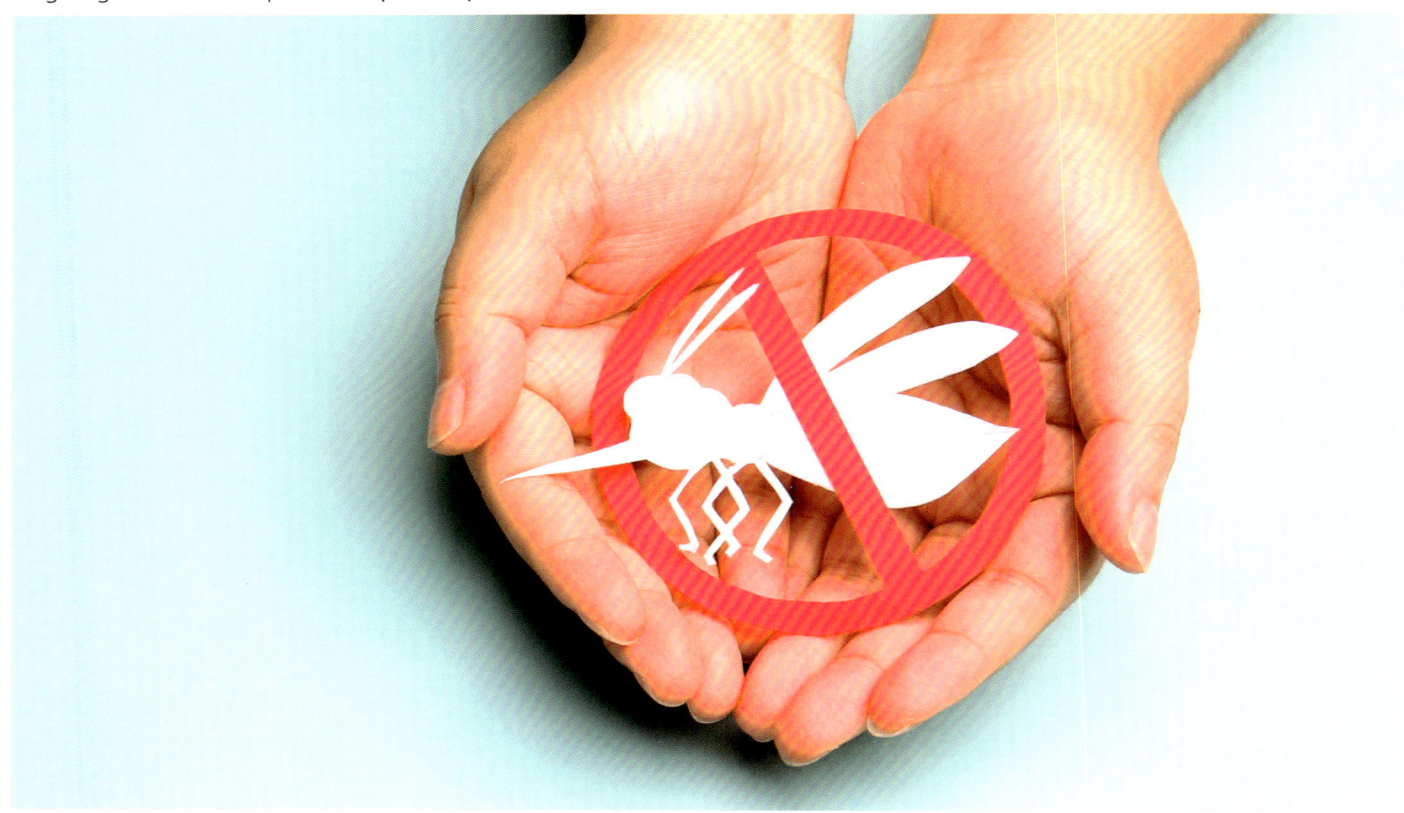

Q&A – Malaria vaccines

For about a century, scientists have been trying to find an effective vaccine against malaria. It has not been easy. There have been about 140 vaccine candidates and, so far, only one – GSK's RTS,S – has been approved for widespread use. From next year, it is hoped, there will be another, named R21, courtesy of Oxford University.

In contrast to a relatively simple virus such as Covid-19, the malaria parasite is highly complex and, crucially, much bigger. 'With malaria there are thousands of potential targets,' says Katie Ewer, professor of vaccine immunology at Oxford's Jenner Institute.

So how does the Oxford vaccine work? Ordinarily, once a mosquito has bitten someone, the malaria parasite travels from their skin through the lymphatic system to the blood and finally to their liver, where it causes the infection that makes them ill.

Many previous vaccines have tried to target the parasite when it is in the blood, but by then, says Ewer, 'that's a very, very tall order.' What R21 does is target the parasite early in its lifecycle, just after a person has been bitten by a mosquito and before they get sick.

'R21 is trying to block the parasites before they get to your liver and set off infection,' says Ewer. 'And that's the mechanism for how it works.

'By targeting the earlier stage of the lifecycle,' she adds, 'there are fewer parasites for the vaccine to mop up, and there's less diversity in the parasite at that stage as well.'

Another British-made malaria vaccine with more modest efficacy levels, GSK's RTS,S, approved by the WHO last year, is poised to be more widely deployed from next year. 'The two leading vaccines in the world for malaria are [from] a UK-headquartered company and a UK university,' Hill said.

'The UK is good at this stuff … It would be tragic if suddenly, as new tools become available, and we can have a real impact – and that's not hard to see now by getting these [vaccines] out there – if we were to just we turn off the taps on funding. And there is a risk of that.'

Gareth Jenkins, director of advocacy at Malaria No More UK, echoed Hill's appeal, saying that 'for new British inventions to achieve their potential, British leadership must continue', starting at the Global Fund conference, to be hosted by the US president, Joe Biden.

'This will be the new PM's first foreign policy test – for the sake of millions of children's lives, global health security and British relations with its closest ally, it's a test she cannot fail,' he added.

Scientists have been trying to find a good vaccine against malaria for about a century, with the first clinical trial taking place in the 1940s. The disease kills hundreds of thousands of people every year, mostly children under five in sub-Saharan Africa.

R21, the first malaria vaccine to meet a WHO efficacy target of 75%, is licensed to the Serum Institute of India. It is ready to manufacture at least 200 million doses annually from next year if the jab is given the green light after results from the wider trial, expected later this year.

Prof Halidou Tinto, regional director of the health sciences research institute (IRSS) in Nanoro, and the Burkina Faso trial principal investigator, said that while production was not expected to be an issue, the big challenge for poor African countries was how to fund the vaccine's rollout. 'This may be … the issue that could delay the deployment,' he said.

The trial in Burkina Faso involved more than 400 children aged between five and 17 months getting three doses of the vaccine in 2019, followed by a single booster shot 12 months later, largely before the peak of the malaria season.

The results, published in the Lancet Infectious Diseases, show that in those children given a booster shot with a higher dose of an immunity-boosting adjuvant the vaccine proved 80% effective. That figure fell to 70% in those who were given a booster with a lower dose of the adjuvant.

No serious side-effects were noted, researchers said.

A spokesperson for the Foreign, Commonwealth and Development Office said: 'As the third largest donor to the Global Fund the UK has invested £4.1 billion to date to fight Aids, tuberculosis, and malaria around the world. We will continue to support its vitally important work.'

7 September 2022

The above information is reprinted with kind permission from *The Guardian*.
© 2023 Guardian News and Media Limited

www.theguardian.com

How climate change is amplifying mosquito-borne diseases

By Alex Jackson, WMP

Mosquito-borne diseases kill more than one million people and infect up to 700 million each year – almost one in ten people. As the planet warms and climate change lengthens the mosquito season, the world's deadliest creature will expand its geographical range to new regions and re-emerge in areas where mosquito numbers had subsided for decades.

Extreme climate and weather patterns such as droughts, heat waves, floods, and rainfall are increasing in severity and regularity across the globe. These provide favourable conditions for mosquitoes to breed and could help spread their viruses to higher latitudes and altitudes.

Climate change also increases mosquito-borne disease risk in less obvious ways, says Dr Katie Anders, an epidemiologist and director of impact assessment at the World Mosquito Program (WMP).

'For example, when households store water in response to drought, this can increase local mosquito breeding sites and disease risk. Land use changes can also drive migration to cities, increasing the population at risk of explosive outbreaks of dengue and other mosquito-borne diseases.'

Widening geographies

Endemic already across sub-Saharan Africa, Southeast Asia and Latin America, mosquito-borne diseases are re-establishing in populations in different parts of the world. The Early Warning System for Mosquito Borne Diseases (EYWA) shows an upward trajectory in Europe, with malaria cases increasing by 62% and dengue, Zika and chikungunya by 700%. Extreme flooding in Germany last year alone saw mosquito numbers swell up to ten times the usual estimates.

Southern Australia is another recent example of mosquitoes expanding to new geographies. The region is currently grappling with its first major outbreak of Japanese encephalitis, a mosquito-transmitted infection more commonly found in rural southeast Asia and the Pacific Islands. Scientists believe climate change has potentially created a 'perfect storm,' allowing the virus to move further south and gain a foothold in the country.

> 'Rising global temperatures are causing an expansion in the areas in which mosquitoes thrive. This puts more communities at risk and makes more months each year favourable to disease transmission in places already prone to mosquito-borne disease.' — Dr Katie Anders
>
> Director of Impact Assessment at the World Mosquito Program

Although there are more than 3,000 mosquito species in the world, most serious diseases such as dengue, chikungunya, Zika and yellow fever are transmitted by just two – *Aedes aegypti* and *Aedes albopictus* (also known as the Asian tiger mosquito). Dengue, the fastest-spreading mosquito-borne virus in the world, is estimated to infect more than 390 million people every year, with more than half of the world's population now at risk.

Global studies

Research teams across the world have studied data on how reducing global warming could save millions of people from mosquito-borne diseases.

One recent study, led by the London School of Hygiene and Tropical Medicine (LSHTM), predicted that more than eight billion people could be at risk of malaria and dengue by 2080. The research found that global temperature rises could lengthen annual transmission seasons by more than a month for malaria and four months for dengue over the next 50 years. These were based on projections of population growth of roughly 4.5 billion over the same period, and a rise in temperature of 3.7°C by 2100.

A *Nature Reviews* paper further reports how increased global connectivity presents unique risk factors for infectious disease spread, allowing pathogens (a microorganism that can cause disease) to travel further and faster than ever before.

However, researchers in Brazil reported other environmental and socioeconomic factors, such as housing development and population growth, complicate predictions of climate change on future disease distribution patterns. Their research, published in *The Lancet Planetary Health*, looked at the association between rainfall patterns and dengue risk, with a notable difference in rural and urban areas. The authors wrote: 'The effects of hydrometeorological events on dengue transmission are dependent on the local social and ecological conditions that determine the types of larval habitat available in the environment, and household water supply and storage practices.'

Researchers have also looked at how climate change has affected the disease carrying capacity of mosquitoes. A review paper in *The Lancet* assessed the influence of temperature and rainfall, overlaying it with human population density data to estimate the reproductive number (R0; the expected number of secondary infections resulting from one infection). Their findings show that the R0 for all arboviral (infections caused by a group of viruses spread by infected arthropods such as mosquitoes and ticks) diseases tracked has increased since 1950-54. The number of infections transmitted by *Aedes aegypti* was 13% higher and for those spread by *Aedes albopictus* 7%.

Effective and sustainable solutions

'We need to use all the tools in the box to combat the growing threat from mosquito-borne diseases,' says Dr Anders. 'This means governments and communities mobilising to control mosquito populations, strengthening disease surveillance

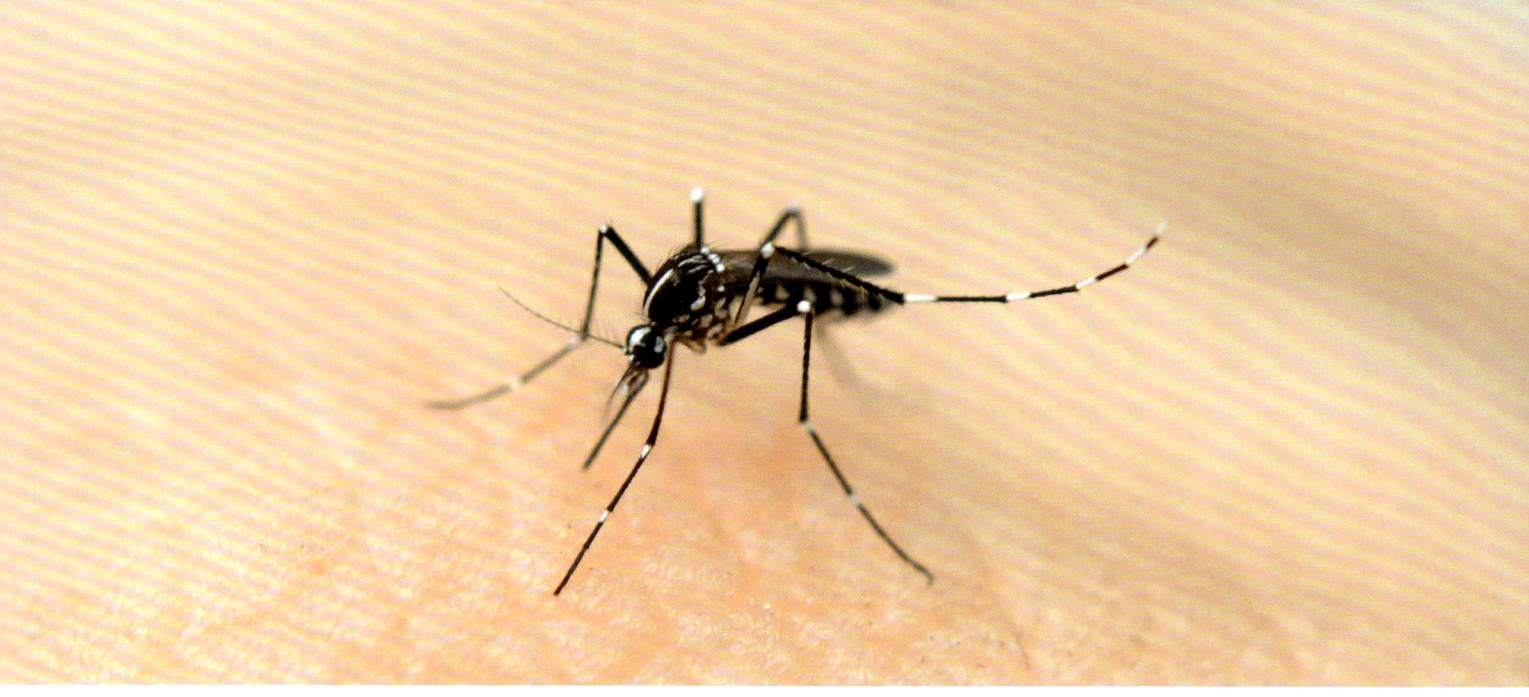

and outbreak response, good clinical management, and rapidly scaling up the delivery of effective interventions like Wolbachia, as well as new dengue vaccines when they are available.'

The urgent need for effective and sustainable strategies to control mosquito-borne disease is reflected in the World Health Organization's (WHO) launch of a Global Arbovirus Initiative on 31 March 2022. The initiative will focus resources on risk monitoring, pandemic prevention, preparedness, detection and response.

Dr Mike Ryan, head of the WHO Emergency Programme, said: 'There is an urgent need to re-evaluate the tools at hand and how these can be used across diseases to ensure efficient response, evidence-based practice, equipped and trained personnel and engagement of communities.'

Many of the methods used to combat mosquito-borne diseases – including both conventional approaches like insecticide spraying and novel techniques such as the release of sterile male mosquitoes – focus on the suppression of mosquito populations, and need to be reapplied regularly to keep mosquito numbers in check. Wolbachia, unlike other measures, is safe for people, mosquitoes, and the environment.

Wolbachia

A common natural bacteria found in about 50% of insects – Wolbachia is introduced in the female *Aedes aegypti* mosquitoes, preventing them from transmitting diseases. The Wolbachia-carrying mosquitoes are then released in areas where mosquito-borne viruses are endemic. As they breed with wild mosquitoes, the number of mosquitoes with Wolbachia grows over time until it remains high and further releases are not needed.

'Wolbachia changes the paradigm for the control of mosquito-borne disease, by reducing the ability of mosquitoes to transmit disease instead of killing them,' says Dr Anders.

'This self-sustaining, safe and cost-effective method gives communities long-term resilience against the multiple diseases transmitted by *Aedes aegypti* mosquitoes.'

This natural Wolbachia method developed by the World Mosquito Program (WMP) is proving highly effective in 11 countries across three continents, protecting almost nine million people so far. In Yogyakarta city (Indonesia), where a 3-year randomised controlled trial was carried out by WMP in partnership with Universitas Gadjah Mada, there was a 77% reduction in dengue incidence and 86% reduction in hospitalisations in Wolbachia-treated communities.

Monitoring outbreaks

Disease surveillance is also another important aspect of combating mosquito-borne diseases. One recent study discovered that through monitoring and identifying the hotspots of dengue, researchers could help create predictive maps for future outbreaks of other diseases such as Zika and chikungunya. They collected data between 2008 to 2020 from cities in southern Mexico and found that there was a 62% overlap of hotspots for dengue and Zika, and 53% for cases of dengue and chikungunya.

In Southeast Asia, the Dengue Forecasting Model Satellite-based System (D-MOSS) gathers satellite data with local insights from partners on the ground about dengue cases, primarily in Malaysia, Sri Lanka and Vietnam. It aims to provide advanced intelligence to government officials in order to control outbreaks. Similarly, NASA scientists are working with local governments and public health officials in the US to help map the locations of disease-carrying mosquitoes and keep communities safe.

Dr Anders emphasises how important it is to understand and predict the rise and spread of mosquito-borne diseases, factoring health-related costs into public policy. As Dr Anthony Fauci, director of the National Institute of Allergy and Infectious Diseases in the US, so gravely put it: 'Any virus that can efficiently infect *Aedes aegypti* also has the potential access to billions of humans.'

The above information is reprinted with kind permission from the World Mosquito Program.
© 2023 Monash University

www.worldmosquitoprogram.org

Antimicrobial resistance now causes more deaths than HIV/AIDS and malaria worldwide – new study

An article from The Conversation.

By Jonathan Cox, Senior Lecturer in Microbiology, Aston University

Antimicrobial resistance is spreading rapidly worldwide, and has even been likened to the next pandemic – one that many people may not even be aware is happening. A recent paper, published in Lancet, has revealed that antimicrobial resistant infections caused 1.27 million deaths and were associated with 4.95 million deaths in 2019. This is greater than the number of people who died from HIV/AIDS and malaria that year combined.

Antimicrobial resistance happens when infection-causing microbes (such as bacteria, viruses or fungi) evolve to become resistant to the drug designed to kill them. This means than an antibiotic will no longer work to treat that infection anymore.

The new findings make it clear that antimicrobial resistance is progressing faster than the previous worst-case scenario estimates – which is of concern for everyone. The simple fact is that we're running out of antibiotics that work. This could mean everyday bacterial infections become life-threatening again.

While antimicrobial resistance has been a problem since penicillin was discovered in 1928, our continued exposure to antibiotics has enabled bacteria and other pathogens to evolve powerful resistance. In some cases, these microbes are resistant even to multiple different drugs. This latest study now shows the current scale of this problem globally – and the harm it's causing.

Global problem

The study involved 204 countries around the world, looking at data from 471 million individual patient records. By looking at deaths due to and associated with antimicrobial resistance, the team was then able to estimate the impact antimicrobial resistance had in each country.

Antimicrobial resistance was directly responsible for an estimated 1.27 million deaths worldwide and was associated with an estimated 4.95 million deaths. In comparison, HIV/AIDS and malaria were estimated to have caused 860,000 and 640,000 deaths respectively the same year. The researchers also found that low- and middle-income countries were worst hit by antimicrobial resistance – although higher income countries also face alarmingly high levels.

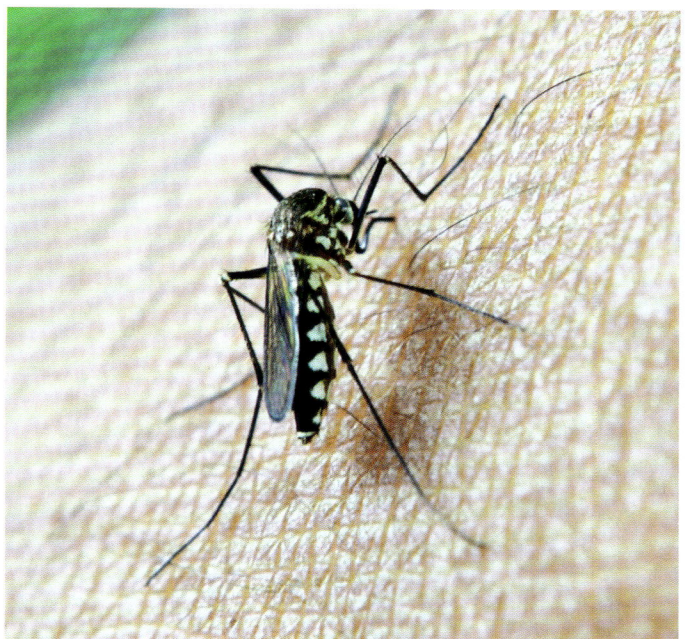

They also found that of the 23 different types of bacteria studied, drug resistance in only six types of bacteria contributed to 3.57 million deaths. The report also shows that 70% of deaths that resulted from antimicrobial resistance were caused by resistance to antibiotics often considered the first line of defence against severe infections. These included beta-lactams and fluoroquinolones, which are commonly prescribed for many infections, such as urinary tract, upper- and lower-respiratory and bone and joint infections.

This study highlights a very clear message that global antimicrobial resistance could make everyday bacterial infections untreatable. By some estimates, antimicrobial resistance could cause 10 million deaths per year by 2050. This would overtake cancer as a leading cause of death worldwide.

Next pandemic

Bacteria can develop antimicrobial resistance in a number of ways.

First, bacteria develop antimicrobial resistance naturally. It's part of the normal push and pull observed throughout the natural world. As we get stronger, bacteria will get stronger too. It's part of our co-evolution with bacteria – they're just quicker at evolving than we are, partly because they replicate faster and get more genetic mutations than we do.

But the way we use antibiotics can also cause resistance.

For example, one common cause is if people fail to complete a course of antibiotics. Although people may feel better a few days after starting antibiotics, not all bacteria are made equal. Some may be slower to be affected by the antibiotic than others. This means that if you stop taking the antibiotic early, the bacteria that were initially able to avoid the effect of the antibiotics will be able to multiply, thus passing their resistance on.

Likewise, taking antibiotics unnecessarily can help bacteria to evolve resistance to antibiotics faster. This is why it's important not to take antibiotics unless they're prescribed, and to only use them for the infection they're prescribed for.

Resistance can also be spread from person to person. For example, if someone who has antibiotic-resistant bacteria in their nose sneezes or coughs, it may be spread to people nearby. Research also shows that antimicrobial resistance can be spread through the environment, such as in unclean drinking water.

The causes driving this global antimicrobial resistance crisis are complex. Everything from how we take antibiotics to environmental pollution with antimicrobial chemicals, use of antibiotics in agriculture and even preservatives in our shampoo and toothpaste are all contributing to resistance. This is why a global, unified effort will be needed to make a difference.

Urgent change is needed in many industries to slow the spread of antimicrobial resistance. Of the greatest importance is using the antibiotics we have smarter. Combination therapy could hold the answer to slowing down antimicrobial resistance. This involves using several drugs in combination, rather than one drug on its own – making it more difficult for bacteria to evolve resistance, while still successfully treating an infection.

The next pandemic is already here – so further investment in research that looks at how we can stop this problem will be key.

20 January 2022

Key Facts

- Antimicrobial resistant infections caused 1.27 million deaths and were associated with 4.95 million deaths in 2019.
- Penicillin was discovered in 1928.
- HIV/AIDS and malaria were estimated to have caused 860,000 and 640,000 deaths in 2019.
- Drug resistance in only six types of bacteria contributed to 3.57 million deaths.
- Antimicrobial resistance could cause 10 million deaths per year by 2050

THE CONVERSATION

The above information is reprinted with kind permission from The Conversation.
© 2010-2023, The Conversation Trust (UK) Limited

www.theconversation.com

What is antimicrobial resistance and why do we need to take action against it?

Antimicrobial drugs are commonly used. We have all heard of antibiotics, which fight bacteria, but there are also antifungals, antivirals and antiparasitics that fight fungi, viruses and parasites, respectively.

The more we use these drugs, the less effective they become and this problem is known as antimicrobial resistance (AMR). It means that microbes have developed resistance to our commonly used medications, meaning these medicines do not always work to treat infections.

What's the problem?

The more we use antimicrobial medicines, the less effective they become against their target organisms, and the less they work at making us better when we need them.

Inappropriate or excessive use of antimicrobials – including antibiotics such as penicillin – allows the target bacteria to develop antimicrobial resistance (AMR). Examples of inappropriate use include taking antibiotics for colds, sore throats, coughs and so on that are viral in origin, so cannot be treated by antibiotics.

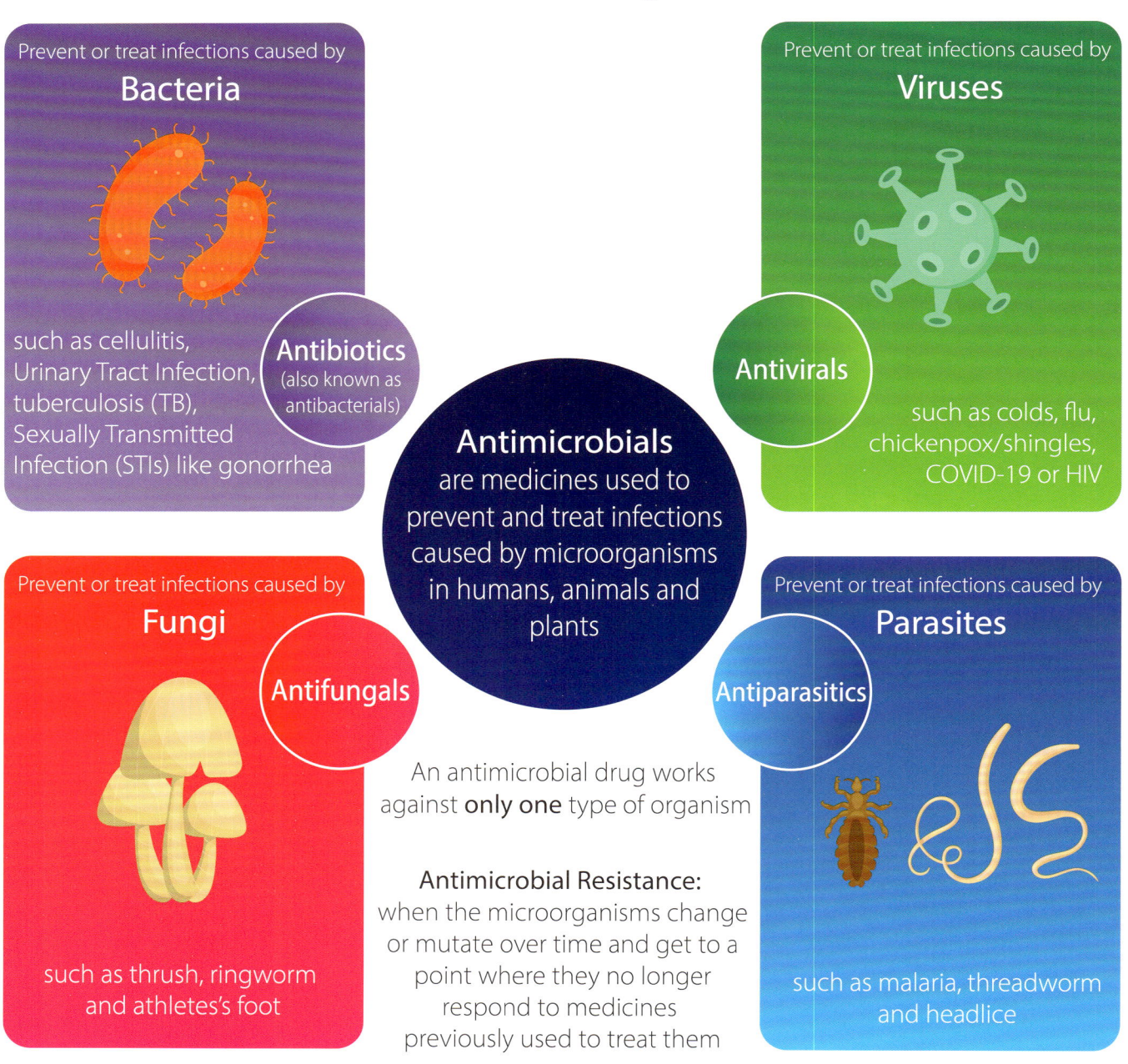

Source: The UK Health Security Agency

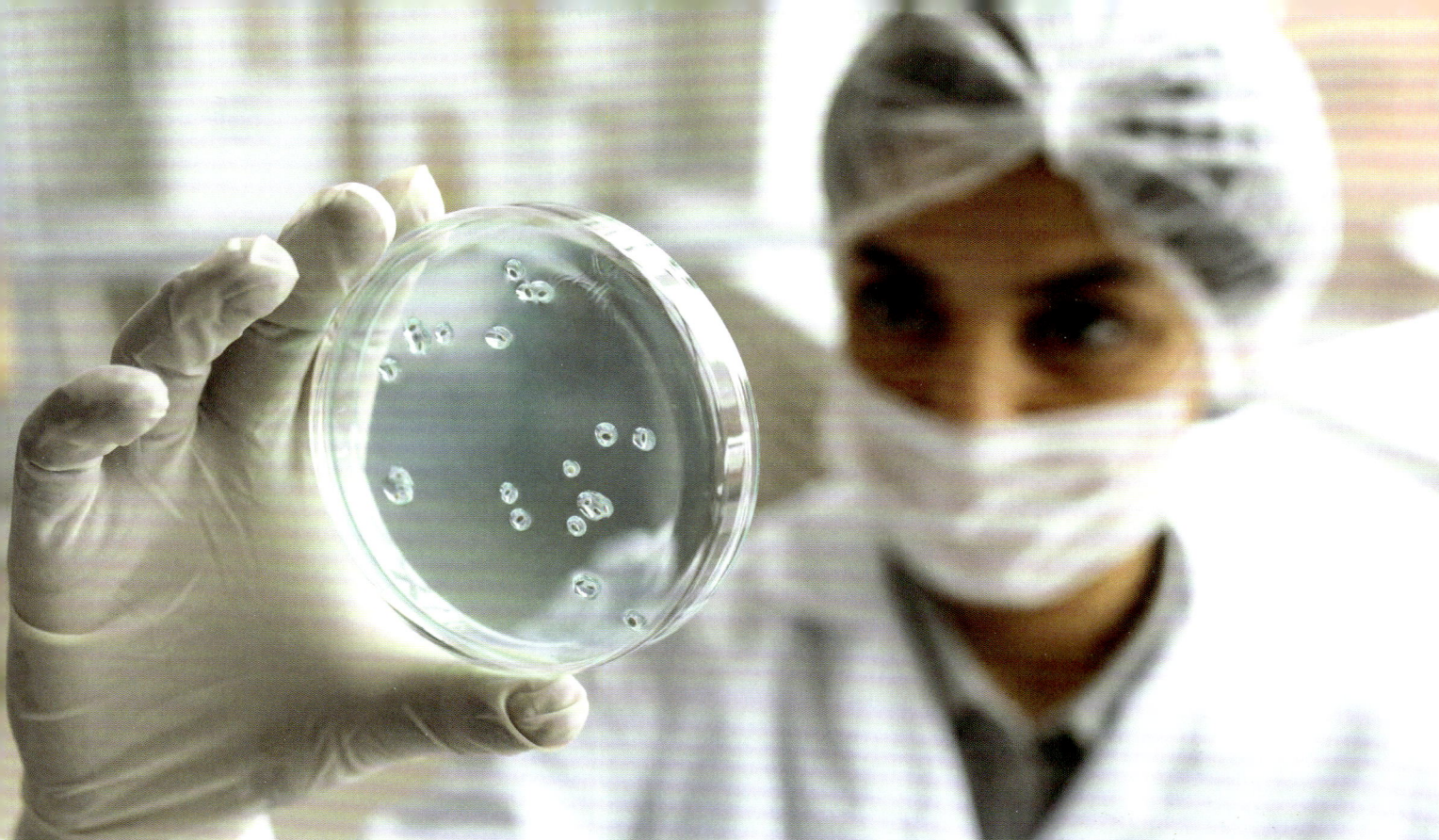

Drug resistant microbes are difficult to treat, and they may be impossible to treat in vulnerable people or people with weak immune systems. Tackling AMR is important for us all, but particularly those who are at higher risk of infection or of getting seriously unwell.

In the absence of effective antibiotics, cancer treatments and common surgeries like caesareans would become very high-risk procedures and for many people, could lead to infections that cannot be treated and may become fatal.

A global review of AMR and its future impact estimated that there would be 10 million global AMR deaths annually from the year 2050 if we do nothing to preserve our current effective antibiotics or do not develop new ones.

AMR also causes problems in settings like hospitals because in some cases, inpatients contract infections known as 'healthcare associated infections' which pose a serious risk to patients, staff and visitors to health and social care sites.

You may have heard the term 'superbug' to describe drug resistant microbes such as Methicillin-resistant Staphylococcus aureus, better known as MRSA. MRSA is a common healthcare associated infection that has developed naturally to resist antibiotics, making infections harder to treat and increasing the risk of disease spread, severe illness and death.

In some countries, problems of sanitation and a lack of clean drinking water can mean infections spread more easily and, in turn, this means drug resistant microbes spread more easily. As COVID-19 has demonstrated, infections do not respect borders. This is a problem that impacts everyone.

The cost of AMR to the economy is significant. Those suffering prolonged illness due to AMR infections are more likely to stay in hospital. The longer the stay in hospital may mean the greater the need for expensive medicines, and the greater the financial impact on the person who is sick.

Spreading awareness, Stopping resistance

Stopping resistance starts with reducing inappropriate prescribing. Antimicrobial medicines should only be taken when a doctor has made a prescription.

Everyone should avoid asking their doctor, nurse, dentist or pharmacist to prescribe antibiotics. And when a health professional prescribes antibiotics, it is important that you always take them as directed, never save them for later and never share them with others.

Healthcare professionals in general practice can also contribute by involving patients in shared decisions about treatments of illnesses, such as delaying prescriptions or offering back-up prescriptions if symptoms do not improve.

17 November 2021

The above information is reprinted with kind permission from the UK Health Security Agency.
© Crown Copyright 2023
This information is licensed under the Open Government Licence v3.0
To view this licence, visit http://www.nationalarchives.gov.uk/doc/open-government-licence/

www.ukhsa.blog.gov.uk

Future Health

Chapter 2

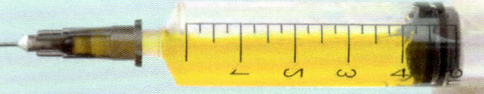

UK 'no better prepared for the next pandemic' with 'dangerous gaps' in its health security

A former Government advisor has warned that the NHS would not survive another deadly new virus, as the Covid-19 inquiry begins on Tuesday.

By Sarah Newey, global health security correspondent

The UK is no better prepared for the next pandemic than it was for the coronavirus, a former top Government scientific advisor has warned.

Ahead of the Covid-19 inquiry – which kicks off on Tuesday with preliminary hearings on Britain's pandemic preparedness and response – academics, Government insiders and industry experts said the country still has 'dangerous gaps' in its health security.

The UK has performed well in several areas, including vaccine development, the agility of regulators and the ONS surveillance programme. But experts are concerned that key infrastructure has been sold or dismantled, that coordination within Whitehall on pandemics is lacking, and that the NHS would not survive another deadly new virus.

'I was one of the people who thought the pandemic would be a great incentive to sort ourselves out,' Professor John Bell, regius professor of medicine at the University of Oxford and a member of the UK's Covid vaccine task force during the pandemic, told the Telegraph.

'It hasn't quite worked out like that, if I'm honest. We did lose hundreds of billions, maybe trillions of pounds, so it was a pretty robust kick. But say we got a transmissible avian flu – or worse, a virus which carried a fatality rate of about 30 or 40 per cent. Would we be ready? I think the answer is absolutely not,' he said.

In particular, experts are critical of the sale of the Vaccine Manufacturing and Innovation Centre in April, a £200-million government-funded centre that aimed to combine vaccine manufacturing and research in one place.

The Government said this was needed to keep the site open, and the takeover by Catalent Biotherapeutics will 'strengthen' the life sciences industry – much like Moderna's decision to build an mRNA vaccine plant in Britain, with almost £400 million of UK funding.

But Professor Rebecca Glover, an assistant professor in infectious disease policy at the London School of Hygiene and Tropical Medicine, called the sale 'short sighted'.

'Dismantling important long-term preparedness infrastructures like the VMIC makes little economic or public health sense,' she said, adding that it gives the Government less flexibility to respond to new threats.

Industry insiders are also concerned that there are gaps in the UK's ability to manufacture new drugs, especially antibody treatments, and that scientific and commercial expertise has not been brought into Whitehall.

In the summer Kate Bingham, who headed the UK's vaccine taskforce, told the *Guardian* she would not return to the role in another pandemic because the Government 'shouldn't be scrambling for people on the outside to come in and help'.

Outbreaks 'more likely' than military invasion

Prof Bell said that he had hoped the pandemic would push the UK to treat health security more like a national security threat, with a clear central command responsible for coordinating any response – especially as this is 'more likely' than a military invasion.

'The government still hasn't operationalised the response to pandemic threats – if the Russians attacked us, we'd turn to the armed forces. Where's the equivalent for pathogens? Governments are increasingly letting pandemic planning fall down the priority list, which is a mistake,' he said.

Adam Bradshaw, a public health analyst at the Tony Blair Institute for Global Change, added: 'Health security is national security. That means being able to manufacture your own medical products – whether vaccines or PPE or therapeutics. It's a small investment now for a massive payoff in the future.'

He said funding cuts for both the UK Health Security Agency and the international aid budget has also hit investment in scientific initiatives across the globe, including disease surveillance. Britain had been a key backer of a 'pandemic radar' at the G7.

'The major lack of funding leaves a major hole,' Mr Bradshaw said. 'Two years ago everyone was saying we'd never underinvest again… that promise has been broken.'

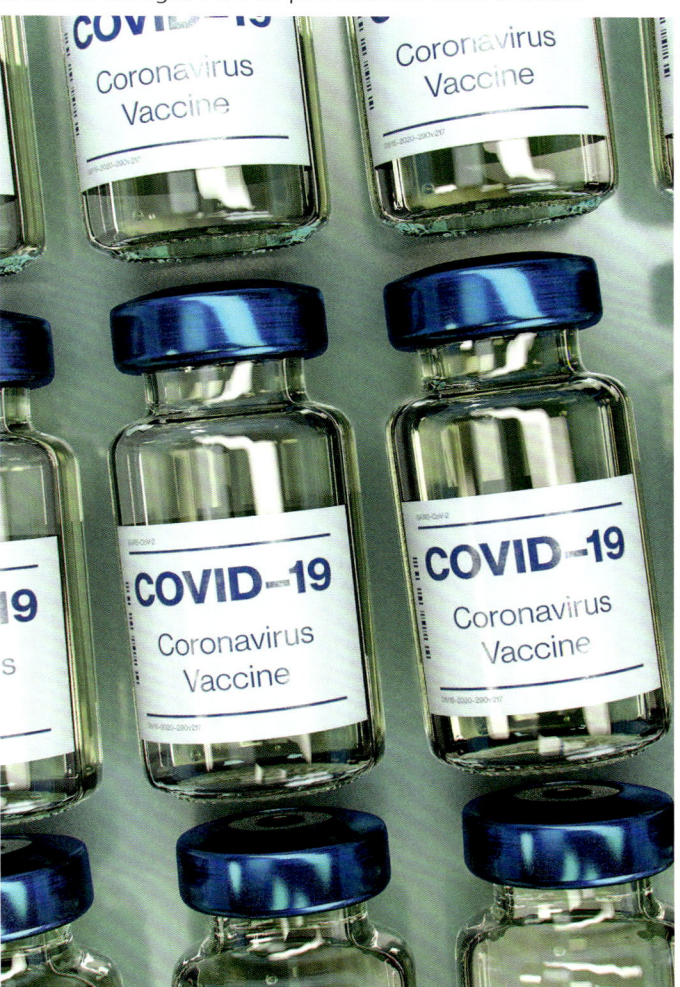

NHS 'is our achilles heel'

Experts are also concerned that the NHS is in a more fragile state than when Covid emerged in early 2020. Even if targets to develop a new vaccine within 100 days of discovering a new pathogen are met, it would be at the forefront of a crisis for three months.

'It is our achilles heel,' said Prof Bell. 'If we got clobbered by a really nasty virus, or a virus with a 30-40 per cent mortality, the health system wouldn't stand up to it.

'I'm normally optimistic, I don't want to be a doom monger. But I think people do need to be aware of the fact that the pandemic we just went through – which has had very large suffering and a very large death toll – was, in pathogen terms, not that bad,' Prof Bell said.

He added that he did think that the UK is better prepared in terms of testing infrastructure – and it was right to roll this back when the acute risk subsided.

Disease surveillance and vaccine development are also areas of strength, while the UKHSA pointed to several initiatives – including the National Variant Assessment Platform, and the new Centre for Pandemic Preparedness – as significant developments.

The first phase of the Covid inquiry, chaired by Baroness Heather Hallett, kicks off on Tuesday in London, after being postponed for two weeks due to the Queen's death. The session is largely procedural, and public hearings will not begin until spring 2023. The first phase will examine Britain's pandemic preparedness and response.

A Government spokesperson said: 'We are committed to learning lessons to inform our preparedness for future pandemics – and the inquiry will be vital in doing this.

'We continue to enhance all aspects of pandemic preparedness nationally and internationally, including spearheading the UK's work to develop a robust and reliable global early warning system to detect new infectious disease threats and keep the public safe.'

4 October 2022

The above information is reprinted with kind permission from *The Telegraph*.
© Telegraph Media Group Limited 2022

www.telegraph.co.uk

How can the world handle the next pandemic if it struggles with new variants?

A better and more modernised approach to preparing for disease outbreaks is crucial to save lives in the future.

By Professor Martin Antonio and Professor Adam Kucharski, Co-Directors of the Centre for Epidemic Preparedness & Response at the London School of Hygiene & Tropical Medicine

March 2022 marks two years since the World Health Organization (WHO) declared the rapid and wide spread of COVID-19 to be a pandemic. It was – sadly – clear that the world wasn't ready.

Two years and more than six million deaths later, and following scores of articles about how countries could have done better, what have we learnt? Are we ready for the next threat?

The Omicron variant has provided an unwanted but useful test, and the results do not bode well for the next pandemic. The response to Omicron has been fragmented, inconsistent and often evidence-free. But despite these problems, there are some examples emerging globally for how we can do better in future – and learning from these lessons will be crucial if we want to be better prepared for the epidemics and pandemics to come.

One ongoing problem for COVID-19 has been poor situational awareness and misguided overconfidence in where the infection really is. Early on, the US was looking at China while infections arrived from Europe and elsewhere. Omicron was identified in Botswana and South Africa, but soon cases were appearing everywhere, even arriving from countries that had not detected the new variant yet. If more countries had the capacity to generate genome sequence data locally and sustainably, and better incentives and structures for sharing data, health outcomes could have been different with alarms raised earlier. Instead, we've seen economy-damaging, scattergun travel bans that have had little or no effect.

The hugely valuable COVID-19 insights produced in countries like South Africa and Uganda reflect a vital new era that we should be accelerating for other pathogens too. We are already seeing valuable progress. Ten years ago, sequencing for Ebola outbreaks was typically done by reactive international teams. But during the recent Guinea outbreak, support instead came from regional expertise in our team in The Gambia. This meant that instead of having to wait for a long cycle of information to feed back to the

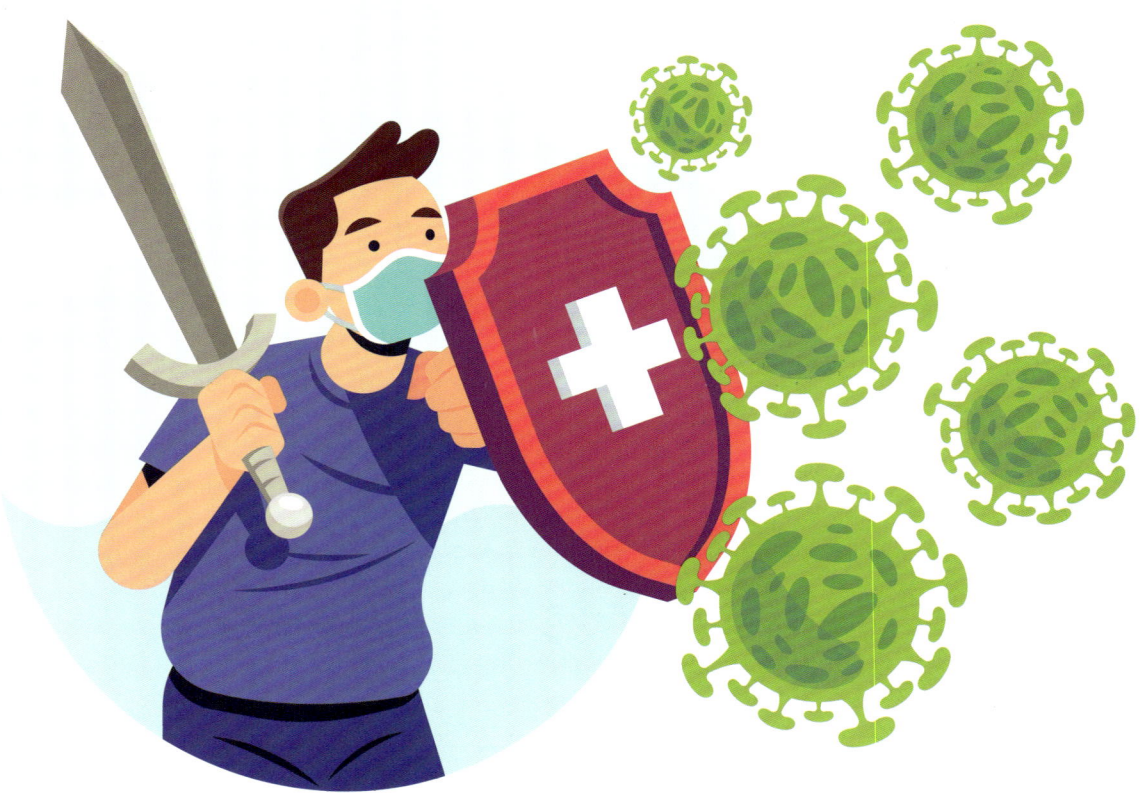

source where people's lives were on the line, the intelligence gathering could be done locally and much more quickly.

To tackle future COVID-19 variants and other pandemics, countries will also need to make better use of the tools that are available. Despite vaccines and rapid tests, several high-income countries introduced lockdowns in response to Omicron. This shows it is not just about having the tools available, it's having the understanding of how to use them effectively. This means considering factors from the dynamics of vaccine confidence to the logistics of deployment and reaching hard to reach populations.

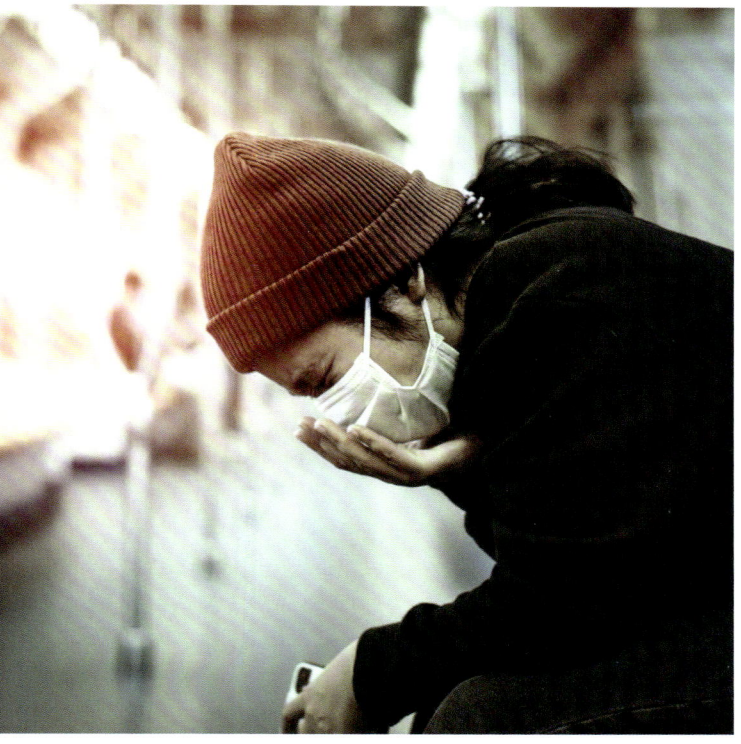

It's about far more than the pathogen itself – it's taking into account people's behaviour, social sciences and breaking down barriers between different disciplines and countries to explore all the complexity that we know impacts on public health and whether interventions are successful or not. It means drawing on lessons from infections like measles, which several European countries have struggled to eliminate despite the availability of a highly effective vaccine.

Omicron has also raised the potential that vaccines may need to be updated in future. We therefore must learn from approaches for tracking evolving viruses like influenza, or the logistics of reactive vaccination campaigns for infections like meningitis. In essence we must open up our minds and draw on the expertise and knowledge that can be found on the ground in all communities impacted by outbreaks. Connecting the dots will make front-line responses much stronger.

Despite the tools now available for COVID-19, resources and expertise are typically concentrated in a relatively small number of countries. The result? A fragmented and introspective international response, one of reactive travel bans and struggling domestic policies.

We need a new approach for this era of pandemics. An approach that is decentralised: a global focus that benefits from local knowledge and expertise. At the London School of Hygiene & Tropical Medicine (LSHTM), we have staff deployed in multiple countries, with the aim of moving beyond reactive research to build longer-term programmes. We need a future where we transition away from a centralised, ad-hoc, fragmented approach to epidemic science to one where crucial methods and capacity are widely available.

To prepare for future pandemics, we will need to identify the best evidence and turn it into the best action. Omicron has revealed the huge gaps that remain within the global response. But globally it also provides an opportunity to learn before the next threat arrives. That means looking beyond Europe and the US, and bringing together the best global evidence on what a good response requires. That is at the heart of LSHTM's new Centre for Epidemic Preparedness & Response.

That is why the Centre will create decentralised fellowships for early career researchers that can be embedded within the places that will have most impact. And that is why we will draw heavily on broader strategic perspectives and expertise from WHO AFRO and other partners at our upcoming launch.

By generating, aggregating and listening to evidence from dozens of countries we can move beyond outdated ways of tackling epidemics – strategies that have fallen tragically short over the last two years.

* Martin Antonio is Professor of Molecular Microbiology & Global Health, based at The MRC Unit The Gambia at LSHTM, and Adam Kucharski is Professor of Infectious Disease Epidemiology at LSHTM.

29 March 2022

Discuss

As a class, discuss whether or not you think travel bans have been effective on the spread of COVID-19 and new variants.

What could be done in future to prevent new variants of COVID-19?

The above information is reprinted with kind permission from the London School of Hygiene & Tropical Medicine.

© 2023 London School of Hygiene & Tropical Medicine

www.lshtm.ac.uk

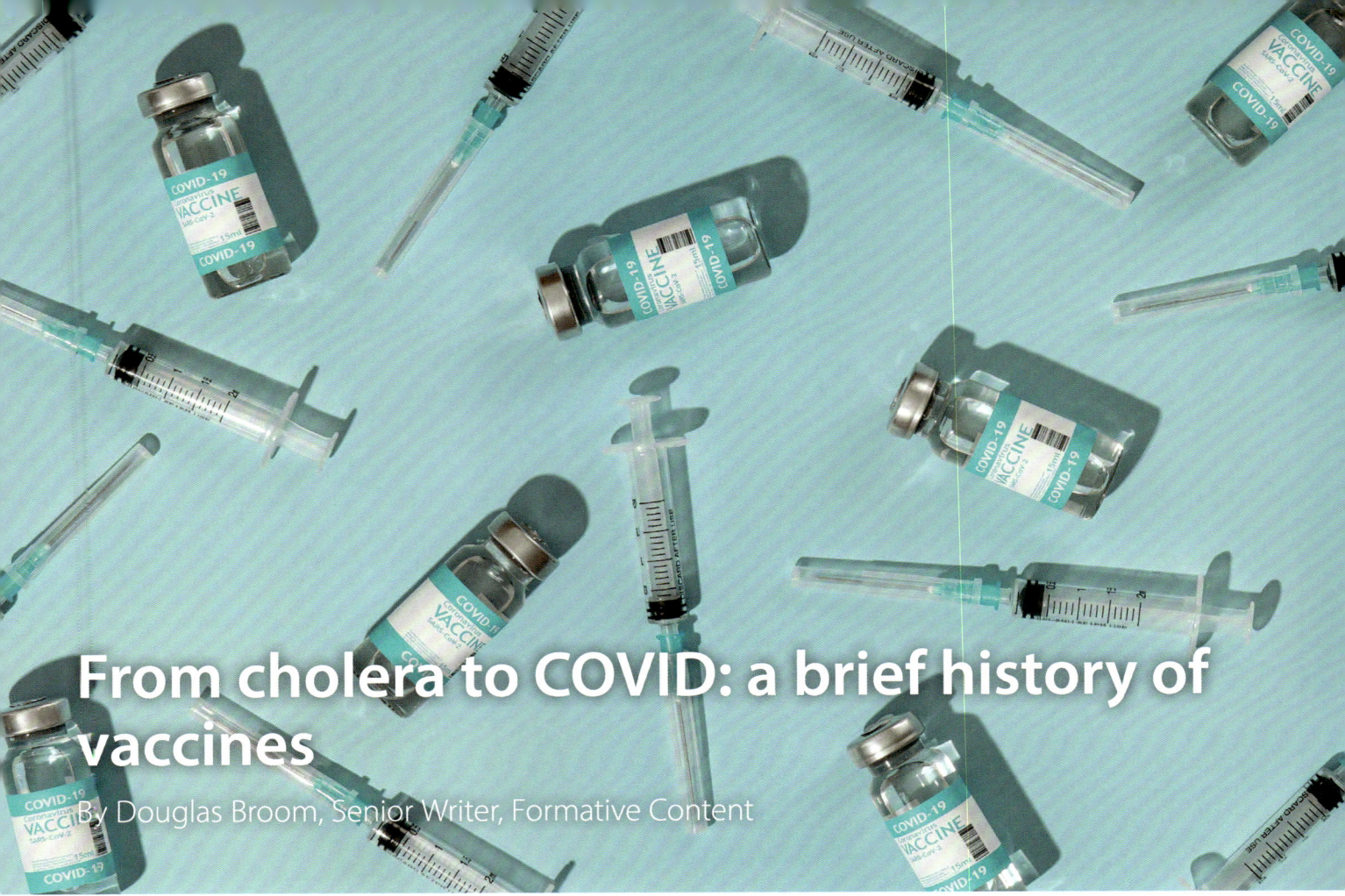

From cholera to COVID: a brief history of vaccines

By Douglas Broom, Senior Writer, Formative Content

The idea of vaccinating people against deadly disease dates back centuries.

Today, vaccines save four million lives every year.

And the COVID-19 pandemic saw the most rapid vaccine development ever.

To mark World Immunization Week, we look back at the history of vaccines.

Every minute, eight children's lives are saved by vaccines, according to the World Health Organization (WHO). Previously fatal diseases like smallpox and polio have been virtually eliminated around the world. But how did this lifesaving breakthrough come about?

The idea of using cells from infectious diseases to stimulate the human body's immune system to fight them is not new. Historians say people were using basic forms of immunization centuries ago.

Vaccines have come a long way since then, with inoculations now available to tackle most of the world's worst infections. The COVID-19 pandemic saw new vaccines developed in record time - ready in just 12 months compared to the usual average of 10 to 15 years.

The remarkable success of vaccines has not been without its challenges - one of the main ones being misinformation and anti-vaccination sentiment, says WebMD, which can be traced back to the 1860s with smallpox immunization fears.

The pandemic also derailed immunization efforts in many countries. The WHO says the suspension of vaccinations in over 68 countries has put at least 80 million children under the age of one at risk.

With studies reporting increasing numbers of cases of measles, diphtheria, polio and dengue and other vaccine-preventable diseases, the WHO has called for the urgent resumption of immunizations across the world.

So, as we mark World Immunization Week, let's look at some of the milestones in the remarkable journey to a vaccine-protected world.

Early forms of vaccinations

As early as the 1500s, people were using simple forms of vaccinations, smearing smallpox on torn skin to create immunity, according to Gavi, the global vaccines alliance.

The process, known as variolation, was recorded as being practised in China in the 17th century and it is said to have cut the death rate from smallpox dramatically. Only around 2% of people died from variolation compared to 30% who caught the disease.

Interest in variolation in North America was sparked by Cotton Mather, a New England Christian minister who read a scientific paper about its use in Turkey. He discovered that one of his servants, who was from what is now Libya, had undergone the procedure.

The history of vaccines
selection of key dates in the development of vaccines

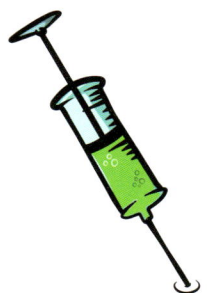

16th century
First mention of **preventative inoculations** in writing in China (smallpox)

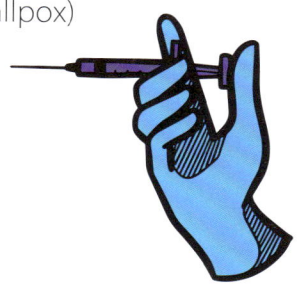

1796
Englishman Edward Jenner introduces the **first scientific method** of vaccination

1853
Smallpox vaccines become **mandatory** in the UK

1885
Frenchman Louis Pasteur develops the **first live virus vaccine** (rabies)

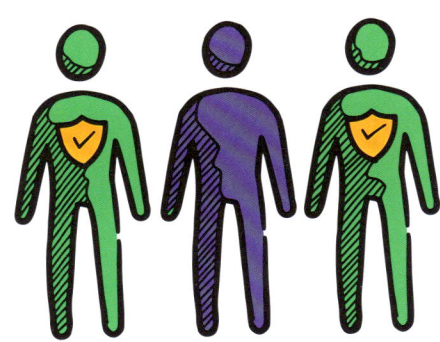

1892-1898
First virus discovered

1920-1926
Development of **tuberculosis, diptheria tetanus and whooping cough** vaccines

1944
First vaccine against the **flu**

1950-1960
First **combination vaccines** (DTP - diptheria tetanus and whooping cough)

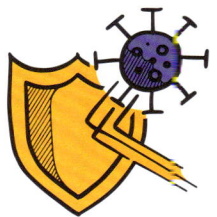

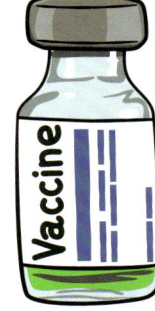

1986
First **genetically engineered vaccine** (hepatitis B)

Source: Statista

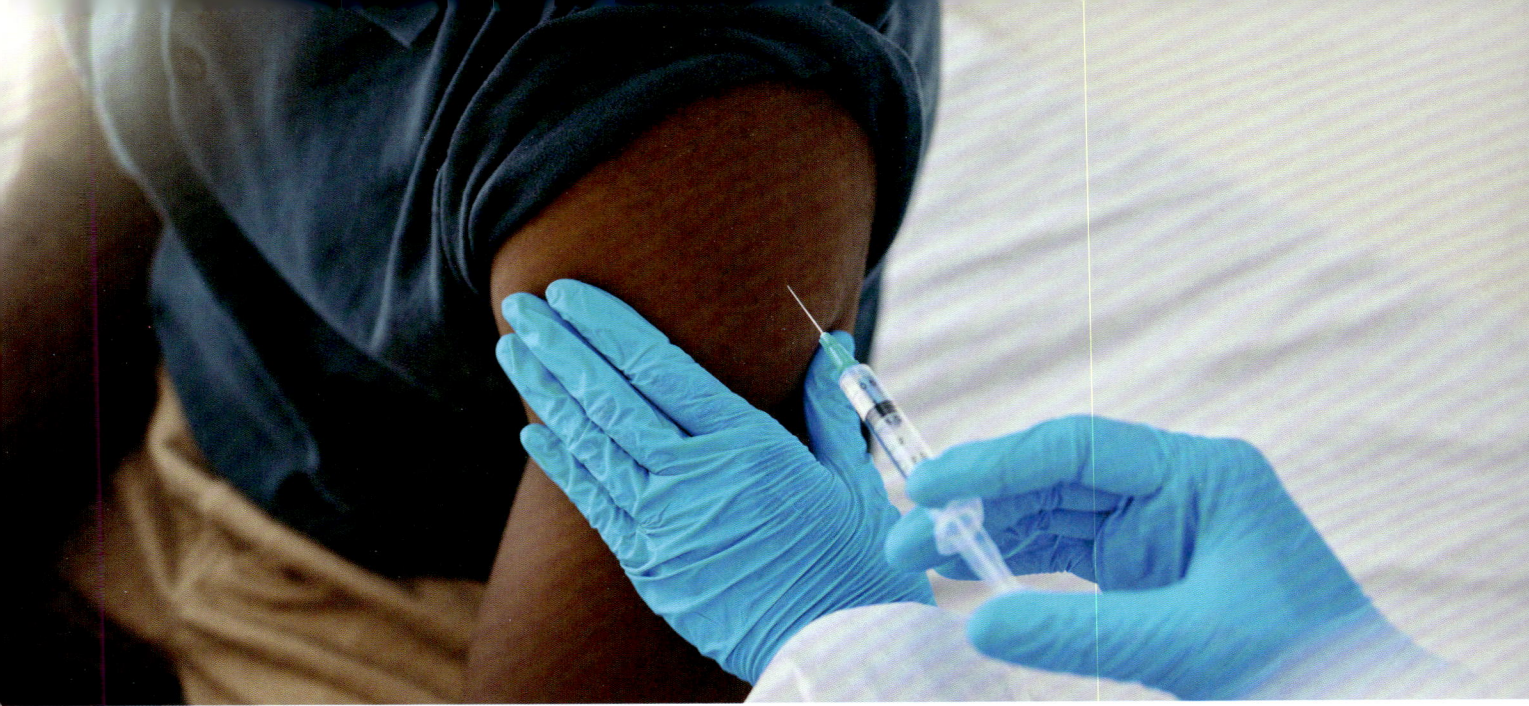

At around the same date, Lady Mary Wortley Montagu, a smallpox survivor and wife of the British ambassador to Constantinople (today's Istanbul), had her three-year-old son inoculated in the city and returned home to promote the benefits of vaccination.

The first modern vaccination

But it was not until 1796 that British country doctor Edward Jenner studied the effects scientifically. Noticing that women working at a local dairy were immune to smallpox because they had already suffered from cowpox, he vaccinated a child with cowpox.

After what historians call the first modern vaccination - named after vaccinia, the Latin name for cowpox - the boy was then exposed to smallpox with no ill effects. For nearly a century afterwards, vaccination meant preventing smallpox.

Laboratory-produced vaccines

Perhaps best-known today for inventing a method of preserving milk, Louis Pasteur discovered a vaccine against chicken cholera in 1879 after mistakenly leaving a vial of the virus open to the elements for a month. Chickens injected with the neglected virus became ill but recovered swiftly.

Pasteur reasoned that the virus had weakened, or attenuated. His accidental discovery opened the door to producing vaccines in the laboratory by creating a less potent form of a virus that would stimulate immunity without harming the patient.

20th-century vaccines

Pasteur went on to develop successful vaccines against anthrax and rabies. In 1885, Spanish doctor Jaime Ferrán created a human cholera vaccine. And in 1896 two German scientists perfected a vaccine against typhoid.

The 20th century saw the creation of vaccines against tuberculosis, tetanus and diphtheria. In 1951, South African virologist Max Theiler won a Nobel prize for a vaccine against yellow fever and in 1955, US scientists announced a successful vaccine against polio.

The eradication of smallpox

In 1967, the WHO set a 10-year target to eliminate smallpox from the world by vaccination. The programme was called Target Zero. By the end of 1970, South America was smallpox-free and the virus was eliminated from Asia by 1975.

In 1977, nearly 200 years after Edward Jenner's pioneering vaccination, Ali Maow Maalin, a 23-year-old hospital cook in Somalia, became the last person to suffer from naturally acquired smallpox. He was vaccinated and survived. In 1980, the WHO declared smallpox eradicated.

The COVID-19 revolution

After the COVID-19 outbreak was confirmed, work began on vaccines at astonishing speed and, within 12 months, new vaccines were being tested and approved. The previous fastest vaccine turnaround was six years for mumps.

The speed was the result of groundbreaking previous work on vaccines for HIV, MERS and SARS, which used RNA and DNA genetic material to stimulate cells to produce 'spike proteins' which create antibodies to fight a virus.

The future of vaccinations

The story of vaccines is far from over. 'Despite rapid advances … in response to COVID-19, more investment is urgently needed in new vaccines and new vaccine technologies,' says Gavi.

'Because, with more than 300 emerging infectious diseases identified since 1940, new pandemic threats lie in the future.'

27 April 2022

The above information is reprinted with kind permission from the World Economic Forum.
© 2022 World Economic Forum

www.weforum.org

Scientists around the world are already fighting the next pandemic

An article from The Conversation.

By David W Graham, Professor of Ecosystems Engineering, Newcastle University & Peter Collignon, Professor of Infectious Diseases and Microbiology, Australian National University

If a two-year-old child living in poverty in India or Bangladesh gets sick with a common bacterial infection, there is more than a 50% chance an antibiotic treatment will fail. Somehow the child has acquired an antibiotic resistant infection – even to drugs to which they may never have been exposed. How?

Unfortunately, this child also lives in a place with limited clean water and less waste management, bringing them into frequent contact with faecal matter. This means they are regularly exposed to millions of resistant genes and bacteria, including potentially untreatable superbugs. This sad story is shockingly common, especially in places where pollution is rampant and clean water is limited.

For many years, people believed antibiotic resistance in bacteria was primarily driven by imprudent use of antibiotics in clinical and veterinary settings. But growing evidence suggests that environmental factors may be of equal or greater importance to the spread of antibiotic resistance, especially in the developing world.

Here we focus on antibiotic resistant bacteria, but drug resistance also occurs in types of other microorganisms – such as resistance in pathogenic viruses, fungi, and protozoa (called antimicrobial resistance or AMR). This means that our ability to treat all sorts of infectious disease is increasingly hampered by resistance, potentially including coronaviruses like SARS-CoV-2, which causes COVID-19.

Overall, use of antibiotics, antivirals, and antifungals clearly must be reduced, but in most of the world, improving water, sanitation, and hygiene practice – a practice known as WASH – is also critically important. If we can ensure cleaner water and safer food everywhere, the spread of antibiotic resistant bacteria will be reduced across the environment, including within and between people and animals.

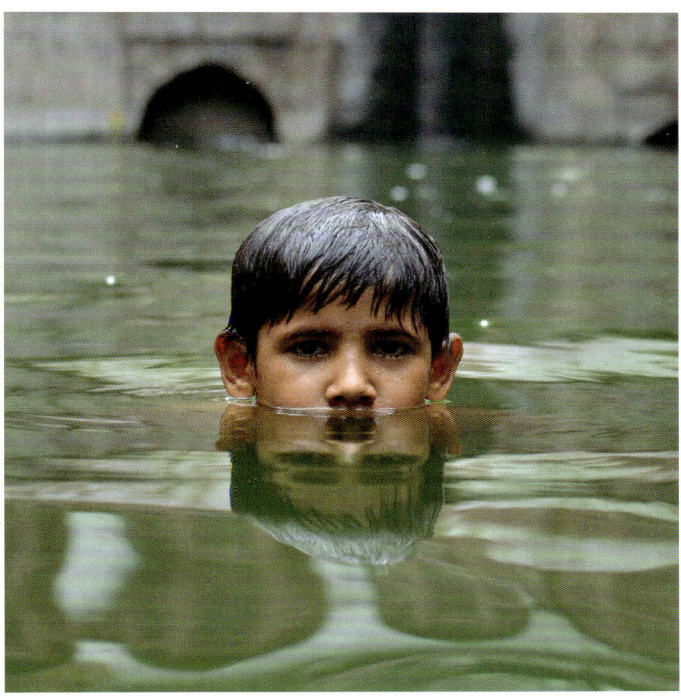

As recent recommendations on AMR from the Food and Agriculture Organization of the United Nations (FAO), the World Organisation for Animal Health (OIE), and World Health Organization (WHO) suggest, to which David contributed, the 'superbug problem' will not be solved by more prudent antibiotic use alone. It also requires global improvements in water quality, sanitation, and hygiene. Otherwise, the next pandemic might be worse than COVID-19.

Bacteria under stress

To understand the problem of resistance, we must go back to basics. What is antibiotic resistance, and why does it develop?

Exposure to antibiotics puts stress on bacteria and, like other living organisms, they defend themselves. Bacteria do this by sharing and acquiring defence genes, often from other bacteria in their environment. This allows them to change quickly, readily obtaining the ability to make proteins and other molecules that block the antibiotic's effect.

This gene sharing process is natural and is a large part of what drives evolution. However, as we use ever stronger and more diverse antibiotics, new and more powerful bacterial defence options have evolved, rendering some bacteria resistant to almost everything – the ultimate outcome being untreatable superbugs.

Antibiotic resistance has existed since life began, but has recently accelerated due to human use. When you take an antibiotic, it kills a large majority of the target bacteria at the site of infection – and so you get better. But antibiotics do not kill all the bacteria – some are naturally resistant; others acquire resistance genes from their microbial neighbours, especially in our digestive systems, throat, and on our skin. This means that some resistant bacteria always survive, and can pass to the environment via inadequately treated faecal matter, spreading resistant bacteria and genes wider.

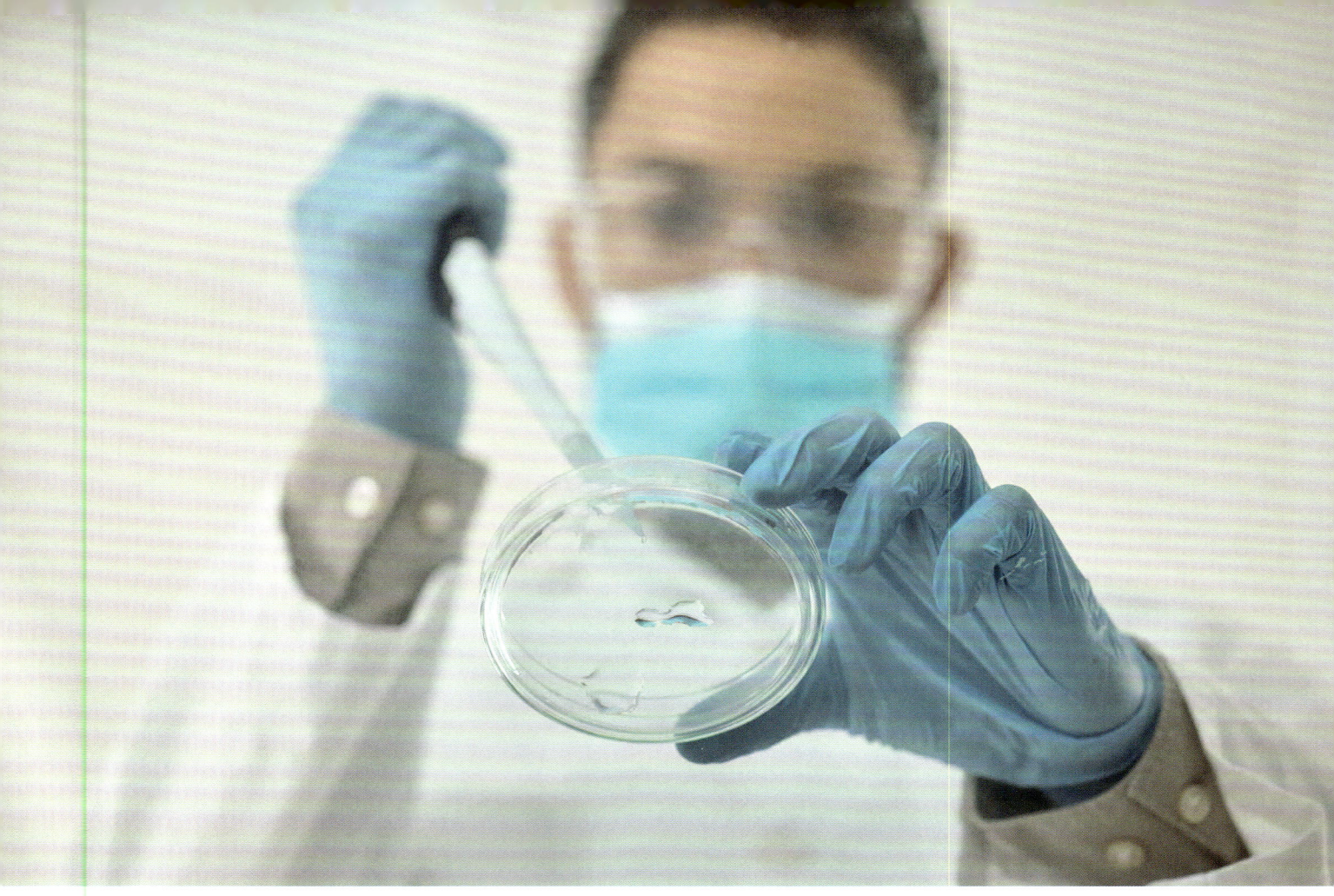

The pharmaceutical industry initially responded to increasing resistance by developing new and stronger antibiotics, but bacteria evolve rapidly, making even new antibiotics lose their effectiveness quickly. As a result, new antibiotic development has almost stopped because it garners limited profit. Meanwhile, resistance to existing antibiotics continues to increase, which especially impacts places with poor water quality and sanitation.

This is because in the developed world you defecate and your poo goes down the toilet, eventually flowing down a sewer to a community wastewater treatment plant. Although treatment plants are not perfect, they typically reduce resistance levels by well over 99%, substantially reducing resistance released to the environment.

In contrast, over 70% of the world has no community wastewater treatment or even sewers; and most faecal matter, containing resistant genes and bacteria, goes directly into surface and groundwater, often via open drains.

This means that people who live in places without faecal waste management are regularly exposed to antibiotic resistance in many ways. Exposure is even possible of people who may not have taken antibiotics, like our child in South Asia.

Spreading through faeces

Antibiotic resistance is everywhere, but it is not surprising that resistance is greatest in places with poor sanitation because factors other than use are important. For example, a fragmented civil infrastructure, political corruption, and a lack of centralised healthcare also play key roles.

One might cynically argue that 'foreign' resistance is a local issue, but antibiotic resistance spread knows no boundaries – superbugs might develop in one place due to pollution, but then become global due to international travel. Researchers from Denmark compared antibiotic resistance genes in long-haul aeroplane toilets and found major differences in resistance carriage among flight paths, suggesting resistance can jump-spread by travel.

The world's current experience with the spread of SARS-CoV-2 shows just how fast infectious agents can move with human travel. The impact of increasing antibiotic resistance is no different. There are no reliable antiviral agents for SARS-CoV-2 treatment, which is the way things may become for currently treatable diseases if we allow resistance to continue unchecked.

As an example of antibiotic resistance, the 'superbug' gene, blaNDM-1, was first detected in India in 2007 (although it was probably present in other regional countries). But soon thereafter, it was found in a hospital patient in Sweden and then in Germany. It was ultimately detected in 2013 in Svalbard in the High Arctic. In parallel, variants of this gene appeared locally, but have evolved as they move. Similar evolution has occurred as the COVID-19 virus has spread.

Relative to antibiotic resistance, humans are not the only 'travellers' that can carry resistance. Wildlife, such as migratory birds, can also acquire resistant bacteria and genes from contaminated water or soils and then fly great distances carrying resistance in their gut from places with poor water quality to places with good water quality. During travel, they defecate along their path, potentially planting resistance almost anywhere. The global trade of foods also facilitates spread of resistance from country to country and across the globe.

What is tricky is that the spread by resistance by travel is often invisible. In fact, the dominant pathways of international resistance spread are largely unknown because many pathways overlap, and the types and drivers of resistance are diverse.

Resistant bacteria are not the only infectious agents that might be spread by environmental contamination. SARS-CoV-2 has been found in faeces and inactive virus debris found in sewage, but all evidence suggests water is not a major route of COVID-19 spread – although there are limited data from places with poor sanitation.

So, each case differs. But there are common roots to disease spread – pollution, poor water quality, and inadequate hygiene. Using fewer antibiotics is critical to reducing resistance. However, without also providing safer sanitation and improved water quality at global scales, resistance will continue to increase, potentially creating the next pandemic. Such a combined approach is central to the new WHO/FAO/OIE recommendations on AMR.

Other types of pollution and hospital waste

Industrial wastes, hospitals, farms, and agriculture are also possible sources or drivers of antibiotic resistance.

For example, about ten years ago, one of us (David) studied metal pollution in a Cuban river and found the highest levels of resistant genes were near a leaky solid waste landfill and below where pharmaceutical factory wastes entered the river. The factory releases clearly impacted resistance levels downstream, but it was metals from the landfill that most strongly correlated with resistance gene levels in the river.

There is a logic to this because toxic metals can stress bacteria, which makes the bacteria stronger, incidentally making them more resistant to anything, including antibiotics. We saw the same thing with metals in Chinese landfills where resistance gene levels in the landfill drains strongly correlated with metals, not antibiotics.

In fact, pollution of almost any sort can promote antibiotic resistance, including metals, biocides, pesticides, and other chemicals entering the environment. Many pollutants can promote resistance in bacteria, so reducing pollution in general will help reduce antibiotic resistance – an example of which is reducing metal pollution.

Hospitals are also important, being both reservoirs and incubators for many varieties of antibiotic resistance, including well known resistant bacteria such as Vancomycin-resistant Enterococcus (VRE) and Methicillin-resistant Staphylococcus aureus (MRSA). While resistant bacteria are not necessarily acquired in hospitals (most are brought in from the community), resistant bacteria can be enriched in hospitals because they are where people are very sick, cared for in close proximity, and often provided 'last resort' antibiotics. Such conditions allow the spread of resistant bacteria easier, especially superbug strains because of the types of antibiotics that are used.

Wastewater releases from hospitals also may be a concern. Recent data showed that 'typical' bacteria in hospital sewage carry five to ten times more resistant genes per cell than community sources, especially genes more readily shared between bacteria. This is problematic because such bacteria are sometimes superbug strains, such as those resistant to carbapenem antibiotics. Hospital wastes are a particular concern in places without effective community wastewater treatment.

Another critical source of antibiotic resistance is agriculture and aquaculture. Drugs used in veterinary care can be very similar (sometimes identical) to the antibiotics used in human medicine. And so resistant bacteria and genes are found in animal manure, soils, and drainage water. This is potentially significant given that animals produce four times more faeces than humans at a global scale.

Wastes from agricultural activity also can be especially problematic because waste management is usually less sophisticated. Additionally, agricultural operations are often at very large scales and less containable due to greater exposure to wildlife. Finally, antibiotic resistance can spread from farm animals to farmers to food workers, which has been seen in recent European studies, meaning this can be important at local scales.

These examples show that pollution in general increases the spread of resistance. But the examples also show that dominant drivers will differ based on where you are. In one place, resistance spread might be fuelled by human faecal contaminated water; whereas, in another, it might be industrial pollution or agricultural activity. So local conditions are key to reducing the spread of antibiotic resistance, and optimal solutions will differ from place to place – single solutions do not fit all.

Locally driven national action plans are therefore essential – which the new WHO/FAO/OIE guidance strongly recommends. In some places, actions might focus on healthcare systems; whereas, in many places, promoting cleaner water and safer food also is critical.

Simple steps

It is clear we must use a holistic approach (what is now called 'One Health') to reduce the spread of resistance across people, animals, and the environment. But how do we do this in a world that is so unequal? It is now accepted that clean water is a human right embedded in the UN's 2030 Agenda for Sustainable Development. But how can we achieve affordable 'clean water for all' in a world where geopolitics often outweigh local needs and realities?

Global improvements in sanitation and hygiene should bring the world closer to solving the problem of antibiotic resistance. But such improvements should only be the start. Once improved sanitation and hygiene exist at global scales, our reliance on antibiotics will decline due to more equitable access to clean water. In theory, clean water coupled with decreased use of antibiotics will drive a downward spiral in resistance.

This is not impossible. We know of a village in Kenya where they simply moved their water supply up a small hill – above rather than near their latrines. Hand washing with soap and water was also mandated. A year later, antibiotic use in the village was negligible because so few villagers were unwell. This success is partly due to the remote location of the village and very proactive villagers. But it shows that clean water and improved hygiene can directly translate into reduced antibiotic use and resistance.

This story from Kenya further shows how simple actions can be a critical first step in reducing global resistance. But such actions must be done everywhere and at multiple levels to solve the global problem. This is not cost-free and requires international cooperation – including focused apolitical policy, planning, and infrastructure and management practices.

Some well intended groups have attempted to come up with novel solutions, but those solutions are often too technological. And western 'off-the-shelf' water and wastewater technologies are rarely optimal for use in developing countries. They are often too complex and costly, but also require maintenance, spare parts, operating skill, and cultural buy-in to be sustainable. For example, building an advanced activated sludge wastewater treatment plant in a place where 90% of the population does not have sewer connections makes no sense.

Simple is more sustainable. As an obvious example, we need to reduce open defecation in a cheap and socially acceptable manner. This is the best immediate solution in places with limited or unused sanitation infrastructure, such as rural India. Innovation is without doubt important, but it needs to be tailored to local realities to stand a chance of being sustained into the future.

Strong leadership and governance is also critical. Antibiotic resistance is much lower in places with less corruption and strong governance. Resistance also is lower in places with greater public health expenditure, which implies social policy, community action, and local leadership can be as important as technical infrastructure.

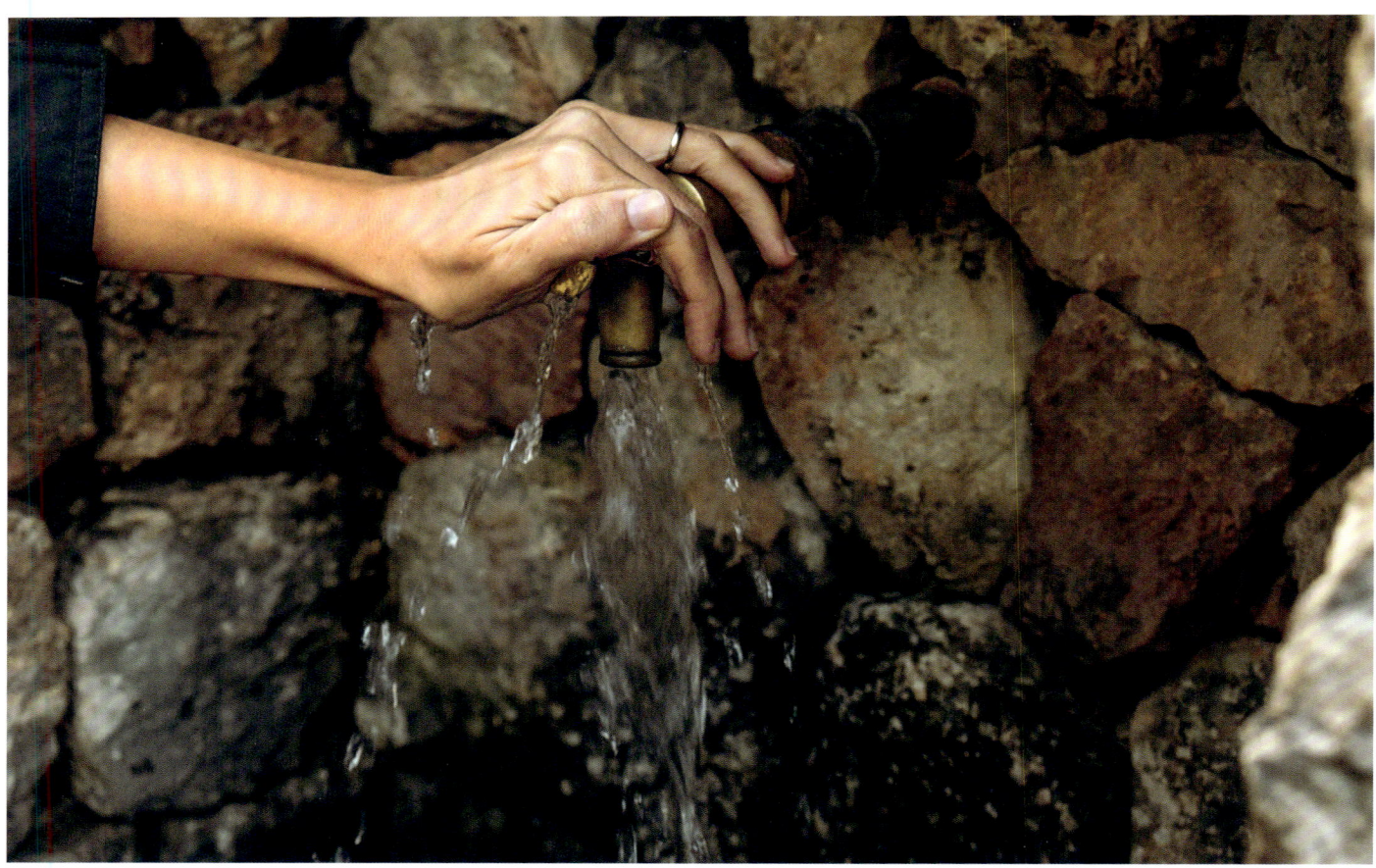

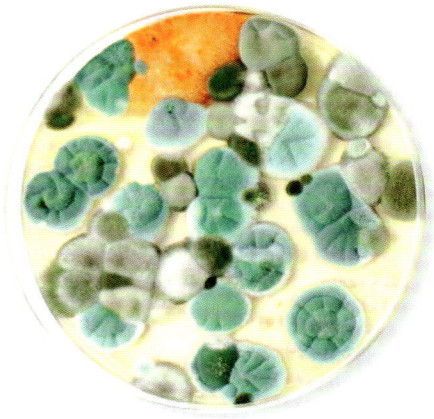
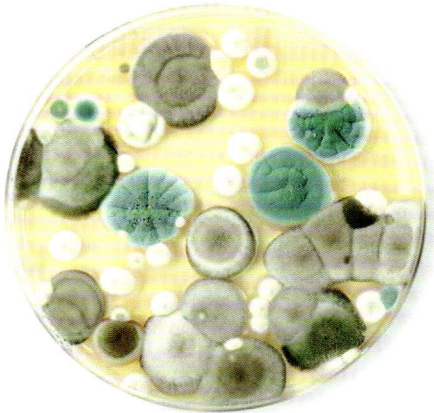
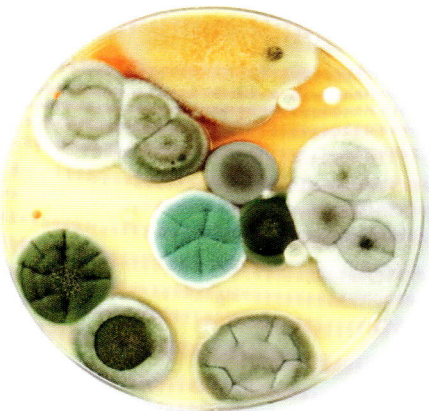

Why aren't we solving the problem?

While solutions to antibiotic resistance exist, integrated cooperation between science and engineering, medicine, social action, and governance is lacking. While many international organisations acknowledge the scale of the problem, unified global action is not happening fast enough.

There are various reasons for this. Researchers in healthcare, the sciences, and engineering are rarely on the same page, and experts often disagree over what should be prioritised to prevent antibiotic resistance – this muddles guidance. Unfortunately, many antibiotic resistance researchers also sometimes sensationalise their results, only reporting bad news or exaggerating results.

Science continues to reveal probable causes of antibiotic resistance, which shows no single factor drives resistance evolution and spread. As such, a strategy incorporating medicine, environment, sanitation, and public health is needed to provide the best solutions. Governments throughout the world must act in unison to meet targets for sanitation and hygiene in accordance with the UN Sustainable Development Goals.

Richer countries must work with poorer ones. But, actions against resistance should focus on local needs and plans because each country is different. We need to remember that resistance is everyone's problem and all countries have a role in solving the problem. This is evident from the COVID-19 pandemic, where some countries have displayed commendable cooperation. Richer countries should invest in helping to provide locally suitable waste management options for poorer ones – ones that can be maintained and sustained. This would have a more immediate impact than any 'toilet of the future' technology.

And it's key to remember that the global antibiotic resistance crisis does not exist in isolation. Other global crises overlap resistance; such as climate change. If the climate becomes warmer and dryer in parts of the world with limited sanitation infrastructure, greater antibiotic resistance might ensue due to higher exposure concentrations. In contrast, if greater flooding occurs in other places, an increased risk of untreated faecal and other wastes spreading across whole landscapes will occur, increasing antibiotic resistance exposures in an unbounded manner.

Antibiotic resistance will also impact on the fight against COVID-19. As an example, secondary bacterial infections are common in seriously ill patients with COVID-19, especially when admitted to an ICU. So if such pathogens are resistant to critical antibiotic therapies, they will not work and result in higher death rates.

Regardless of context, improved water, sanitation, and hygiene must be the backbone of stemming the spread of AMR, including antibiotic resistance, to avoid the next pandemic. Some progress is being made in terms of global cooperation, but efforts are still too fragmented. Some countries are making progress, whereas others are not.

Resistance needs to be seen in a similar light to other global challenges – something that threatens human existence and the planet. As with addressing climate change, protecting biodiversity, or COVID-19, global cooperation is needed to reduce the evolution and spread of resistance. Cleaner water and improved hygiene are the key. If we do not work together now, we all will pay an even greater price in the future.

9 June 2020

THE CONVERSATION

The above information is reprinted with kind permission from The Conversation.
© 2010-2023, The Conversation Trust (UK) Limited

www.theconversation.com

Useful Websites

www.advisory.com

www.independent.co.uk

www.lshtm.ac.uk

www.medicalnewstoday.com

www.medicalnewstoday.com

www.mobilemalaria.com

www.targetmalaria.org

www.telegraph.co.uk

www.theconversation.com

www.theguardian.com

www.ukhsa.blog.gov.uk

www.weforum.org

www.who.int

www.worldatlas.com

www.worldmosquitoprogram.org

Absolute poverty
Inability to meet even the most basic survival needs. This includes the necessities such as food, water, shelter, clothing and health care.

AIDS
Acquired Immune Deficiency Syndrome. AIDS is a potentially fatal illness. It develops at the most advanced stage of HIV.

Air pollution
Air pollution can cause both short-term and long-term effects on health and many people are concerned about pollution in the air that they breathe. These people may include people with heart or lung conditions, or other breathing problems, whose health may be affected by air pollution.

Antibiotic resistance
When an antibiotic has been used a lot, it can lose its ability to kill bacteria – the bacteria become 'resistant' to it.

Antimicrobial resistance
A broad term used to refer to 'drug resistance' where a microbe or virus becomes resistant or immune to the drugs used to treat it. Doctors are increasingly concerned that over-prescription of antibiotics has led to some people developing a resistance which means the drugs are less effective.

Cholera
An infectious disease that affects the small intestine. Cholera is usually contracted from infected water supplies and causes extreme sickness and diarrhoea.

Communicable diseases
Diseases that you can catch from another person or being. Also known as 'infectious' diseases.

COVID-19
Coronavirus disease (COVID-19) is an infectious disease caused by the SARS-CoV-2 virus. First emerging in December 2019 in Wuhan, China, the World Health Organization (WHO) declared a pandemic in March 2020.

Drug
A chemical that alters the way the mind and body works. Legal drugs include alcohol, tobacco, caffeine and prescription medicines taken for medical reasons. Illegal drugs taken for recreation include cannabis, cocaine, ecstasy and speed. These illegal substances are divided into three classes – A, B and C – according to the danger they pose to the user and to society (with A being the most harmful and C the least).

Ebola
An infectious and usually fatal disease that is characterised by severe fever and internal bleeding. It is spread through contact with infected bodily fluids.

Endemic
Native or restricted to a particular place.

Epidemic
Widespread occurrence of an infectious disease.

Glossary

Immune system
The immune system is made up of cells, tissue and organs that protect the body from viruses and infections. The HIV virus attacks the immune system and prevents the body from protecting itself.

Immunisation
Immunisation is the process whereby a person is made immune or resistant to an infectious disease, typically by the administration of a vaccine.

Life expectancy
The average period that a person may be expected to live.

Long-Term Condition
A medical condition that cannot be cured but can be eased or controlled with medication.

Malaria
A life-threatening disease caused by a parasite that is transmitted by Anopheles mosquito. With correct medication and precautions, Malaria is preventable and treatable. Only the female Anopheles mosquito can transmit the disease to a human.

Malnutrition
Malnutrition essentially means 'poor nutrition'. There are two types of malnutrition: undernutrition (when a person's diet is lacking in nutrients and sustenance they need) and overnutrition (when a person's diet is getting far too many nutrients for the body to cope with). Malnutrition can affect anybody, although it tends to be more common in developing countries where there are shortages of food.

NHS
The National Health Service provides free medical care to citizens of England, Scotland, Wales and Northern Ireland.

Non-communicable diseases (NCDs)
These diseases cannot be transmitted from person to person, e.g. heart disease.

Pandemic
A pandemic is an epidemic of disease that has spread across a large region; for instance, multiple continents, or even worldwide.

Poverty
Peter Townsend offers this definition of poverty: 'Individuals, families and groups in the population can be said to be in poverty when they lack the resources to obtain the types of diet, participate in the activities, and have the living conditions and amenities which are customary, or are at least widely encouraged and approved, in the societies in which they belong.' .

Sanitation
Usually refers to access to clean drinking water and adequate sewage facilities. Sanitation is the disposal of human sewage. Inadequate sanitation within a community can lead to disease and polluted drinking water.

Sepsis
Sepsis is a serious complication of an infection. Without quick treatment, sepsis can lead to multiple organ failure and death.

Sexually transmitted disease
A disease or infection that is transmitted through the exchange of bodily fluids such as semen or genital fluids.

Superbug
'Superbug' is a term used to describe strains of bacteria that are resistant to the majority of antibiotics commonly used today.

Tuberculosis (TB)
A bacterial infection spread through inhaling tiny droplets from the coughs or sneezes of an infected person. This is a serious condition but can be cured with proper treatment. Symptoms include a persistent cough, weight loss, night sweats and high temperature.

Vaccine
Vaccines can be prophylactic (example: to prevent or ameliorate the effects of a future infection by a natural or 'wild' pathogen), or therapeutic (e.g. vaccines against cancer are being investigated). The administration of vaccines is called vaccination.

Vector-borne diseases
Diseases that are transmitted among humans or animals, usually by insects. Malaria is an example of a vector-borne disease because it is transmitted by mosquitoes.

World Health Organization (WHO)
WHO is an agency of the United Nations (UN) that is dedicated to global public health issues.

Zika virus
Zika virus disease is mainly spread by mosquitoes. For most people it's a very mild infection and isn't harmful. But it may be more serious for pregnant women, as there's evidence it causes birth defects – in particular, abnormally small heads (microcephaly). Zika doesn't naturally occur in the UK, however cases in the UK are associated with travel to countries or areas with active Zika virus transmission.

Zoonotic diseases
Diseases spread between animals and humans, e.g. rabies.

Index

A
access, to health care 1–2
adolescents, death rate and safety 3
AIDS (Acquired Immune Deficiency Syndrome) 7, 26, 42
air pollution 1, 42
antibiotic resistance 37–41, 42
    see also antimicrobial resistance (AMR)
antibiotics 26–29
    see also antimicrobial resistance (AMR)
antifungals 28
antimicrobial resistance (AMR) 3, 26–29, 42
antiparasitics 28
antivirals 28
antonine plague 6

B
bacteria 26–28, 37
Black Death 5, 6
bubonic plague 5

C
cholera 5, 6–7, 36, 42
climate change 24
climate crisis 1
coccidioidomycosis 4
coronavirus 4, 5, 12
    see also COVID-19
COVID-19 4–13, 29, 42
    impact on global health 8–11
    inquiry 31
    symptoms 12
    variants 32–33
cowpox 36

D
dengue fever 4, 24
diet, unsafe food 2
drug, definition 42

E
ebola virus 4, 15–18, 42
endemic diseases 4, 5
epidemic diseases 4, 5

F
food, unsafe 2
fungi 28

G
global warming 1

H
health care 11
    access 1–2
    equity 1–2
    sanitation 3
health workers 3
hepatitis B 4
HIV (human immunodeficiency viruses) 5, 7, 26

I
immune system 5, 34, 43
immunisation 6, 34, 43
    see also vaccines
infectious diseases 1, 2, 42
influenza 1918 5, 7
influenza H3N2 1968 7

L
life expectancy 11

M
malaria 4, 19–24, 26, 43
malnutrition 1, 11, 43
Methicillin-resistant Staphylococcus aureus (MRSA) 29
Middle East respiratory syndrome (MERS) 12, 13
monkeypox 14
mosquito-borne diseases 24–25
    see also dengue fever; malaria

O
obesity 11
opioids 4
overcrowding 8, 10

P
pandemics 4–7, 30–33, 37
parasites 28
Pasteur, Louis 36
pollution 37, 39
    air 1, 42
poverty 37, 42, 43
public trust 3

R
Russian flu 1889 7

S
sanitation 3, 38–40, 43
sepsis 43
severe acute respiratory syndrome (SARS) 5, 7, 12, 13
smallpox 6, 34–36
Spanish flu see influenza 1918
superbugs 29, 37–39, 43
    see also antimicrobial resistance (AMR)
swine flu 5

T
technology 3
tobacco use 11
tuberculosis (TB) 11, 22, 35, 36, 43

U
unsafe food 2

V
vaccines 2, 22–23, 34–36, 43
vector-borne diseases 43
vulnerable populations 9–10

W
war and conflict, and health care access 1
World Health Organization (WHO)
    urgent health challenges 1–3
    World Malaria Report 19

Z
Zika virus 4, 43
zoonotic diseases 5, 43